Wakefield Press

AN EVERYONE STORY

Duncan McKellar is a psychiatrist who specialises in the care of older people. In 2017 he was a co-author of Australia's landmark Oakden Report, which triggered the Australian Royal Commission into Aged Care Quality and Safety. Most recently he lived in Edinburgh, exploring his Scottish heritage, before returning home to Australia in 2024. He is the co-creator of *A Box of Memories*, a musical written with his daughter Erin, about a family dealing with dementia.

Praise for *An Everyone Story*

'Duncan McKellar's *An Everyone Story* is a book that won't leave your hands or your heart. It profoundly crystallises what happens when our systems become dehumanised and how earnestly we must reach out to mend those all-too-easily neglected. As a filmmaker who's experienced the joys and challenges of sharing our lived dementia experience with the world, I know the immense value that difficult words shared can bring. This book will inspire you to be a better, more grateful human.' – Jason van Genderen, award-winning filmmaker, *Everybody's Oma*, advocate for people with dementia and their carers

'Sitting at the heart of health and social care is empathy and love – the ability to feel with others and to offer care that respects every aspect of their humanity. When people, organisations and systems lose empathy and love, it is disastrous for everyone. In this personal, moving and very important book, Duncan McKellar narrates a powerful story of organisational breakdown and the impact that such failures have on the most vulnerable members of our communities. It is a story filled with sadness but also tinged with powerful hope that, even in the midst of devastation, those who seek the humanness of others can find it.' – Reverend Professor John Swinton, King's College, University of Aberdeen, Chaplain to His Majesty, King Charles III, in Scotland

'An emotional roller-coaster that takes the reader on a journey of courageous and authentic change. Whether we are healthcare professionals, leaders, or just ordinary people hopeful of enabling positive humanity to prevail, Duncan McKellar's exploration of the transformation from toxic to flourishing culture is a humbling reminder of the importance of building compassionate, person-centred, and story-informed lives, where, through collaborative action, we learn to listen to the people we serve. Essential reading.' – Professor Kim Manley CBE, Universities of Christchurch, Canterbury and East Anglia

'A compelling read – like a gripping novel but completely true, and brimming with heartfelt stories. It offers an insider view of dealing with change when there is a massive need, but not everyone is on the same page. I found myself deeply moved, with great respect for the resilience of the author and his colleagues as they responded to profound organisational dysfunction and discovered a more humane way to work. This inspiring story demonstrates the importance of advocacy, commitment, and belief in what one is doing. It is a must-read for people in all caring professions, for politicians, people in the media, people touched by dementia and all causes of human struggle. It is a story for everyone.' – Professor Sue Kurrle AO, consultant for ABC TV's *Old People's Home for 4 Year Olds*

'Duncan McKellar is a skilful and sensitive storyteller who shares his human vulnerability with the understanding that this is something common to us all. It can be confronting to read about what happens when we fail to act rightly toward others, especially people in need – but change is possible, and Duncan provides the reader with insight and tools to help make this happen. This should be required reading for everyone in health, aged and social care, and anyone committed to compassionate leadership. Indeed, compassion and hope are at the heart of this book.' – Associate Professor Colm Cunningham, Executive Director International, HammondCare

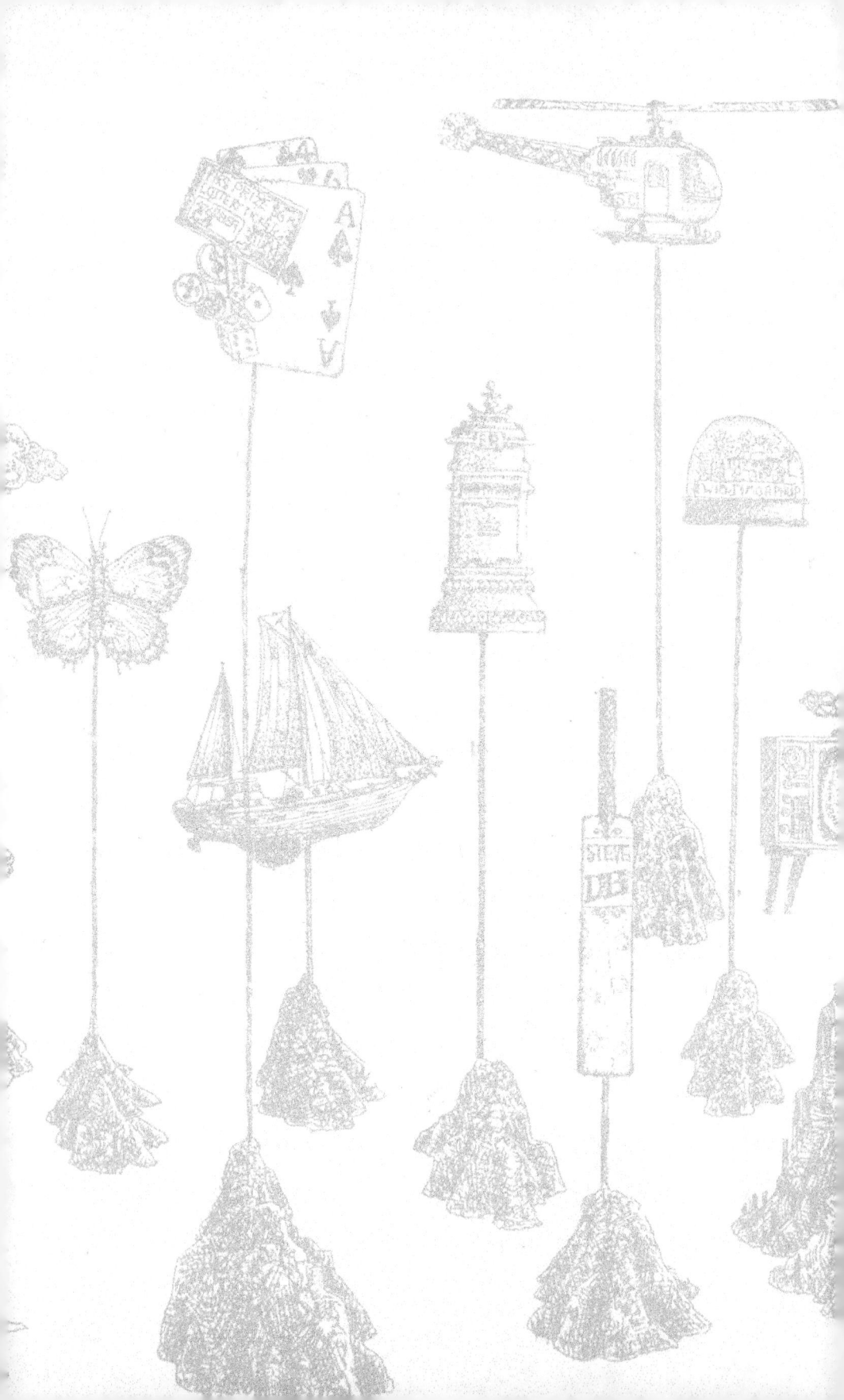

AN EVERYONE STORY

*Finding our way back to compassion,
hope and humanity*

Duncan McKellar

Wakefield
Press

Wakefield Press
16 Rose Street
Mile End
South Australia 5031
www.wakefieldpress.com.au

First published 2024

Cover designed by Stacey Zass
Front cover illustration by Leon Pericles
Edited by Julia Beaven, Wakefield Press
Typeset by Michael Deves, Wakefield Press

ISBN 978 1 92304 217 9

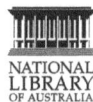

NATIONAL
LIBRARY
OF AUSTRALIA

A catalogue record for this
book is available from the
National Library of Australia

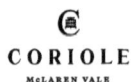

CORIOLE
McLAREN VALE

Wakefield Press thanks
Coriole Vineyards for
continued support

Contents

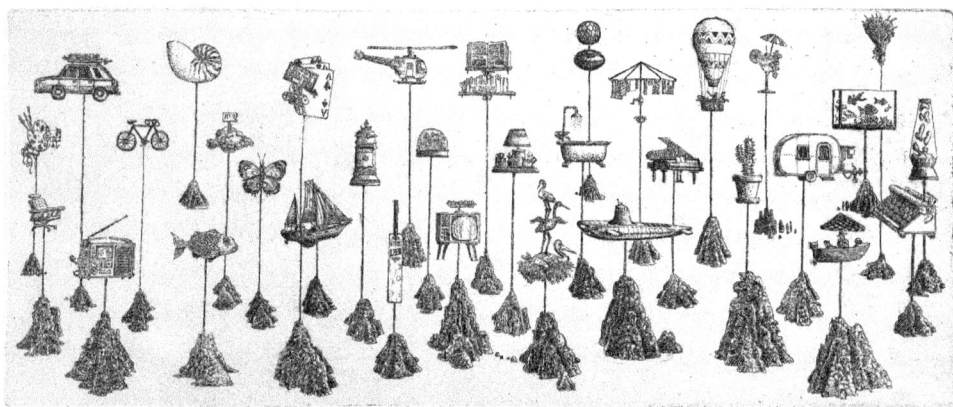

Islands of Lost Memories (2022)
Line etching, 19 x 57 cm
by Leon Pericles AM
Courtesy of the artist

Leon Pericles' *Islands of Lost Memories*

Leon Pericles AM is a treasured Australian artist whose work is acclaimed nationally and internationally, being held in numerous major public and private collections. He works across genres, including painting, printmaking, mixed media and sculpture. The line etching *Islands of Lost Memories*, featured on the cover, poignantly references Leon's experience with his beloved wife, Moi, living with dementia. The image depicts memories, characterised as objects and ideas of personal and sentimental value, gathered from a person's life and transferred between generations, and tethered to earth by the love and strength of others, preventing them from floating away. The tethering of memories reflects the holding of stories that capture the essence of loved people's lives in the wake of change, vulnerability and loss.

The etching is available for purchase from www.leonpericles.com.au in support of the work of Dementia Australia.

Foreword

When Bob, my husband and best friend of forty-six years, suffering from complex and distressing symptoms caused by Lewy body dementia and Capgras syndrome, was transferred to the Oakden Older Persons' Mental Health Service, my family and I were assured that this was where his needs would be best met. Although our first impression was that the buildings and facilities were more run-down than we had expected, we, like most people, trusted that the South Australian Department of Health would provide Bob with the best and most enlightened care available.

It did not take us long to realise that our trust was misplaced.

Bob's experiences at Oakden – the lack of understanding of the effects of his condition, the lack of empathy, and the lack of respect for his individuality and dignity – were horrific for him and extremely distressing for us, his family. The impact of this would dominate our lives for the months and years ahead as we, together with the families of other people with similar experiences, fought for recognition that there was a serious problem, and that action was required to ensure that no older person, living with dementia, or a mental illness, and their families, would have to endure what we did.

Navigating our way through the health and aged care systems was like trying to find our way through a labyrinth. Roadblocks continually appeared, and it seemed like this occurred in the anticipation that we would grow weary, become discouraged and give up.

We refused to do so and, after months of appearing to get nowhere, people started to listen, the press became interested, public awareness increased, and the government was compelled to acknowledge the issues. Eventually, of course, the Australian Royal Commission into Aged Care Quality and Safety was announced, which provided a once-in-a-lifetime opportunity to bring about change in a broken system, although there remains unfinished business.

I have known Duncan McKellar since we met at the time of my family's interview with the Oakden review panel – he provides an account of that conversation in the pages of this book. I greatly respect Duncan's leadership and contribution to the task of bringing about desperately needed reform in the system providing care for older people with complex needs. I am very pleased that he has decided to tell the Oakden story from his perspective, and to place it within the context of his personal story and the broader issues facing our health and social care systems – and how we work together as people. It is a story that needs to be told.

I have been called a 'whistleblower' – but that is not how I see myself. Our family's experience was not isolated and, as you will read, there are many other courageous, although troubling, stories. What kept me going was the hope that no one else would have to go through what we experienced.

Each of us has a voice to use and a story to tell. Regardless of our background, education, or how anxious we might feel, we should not be deterred from coming forward and speaking up about things we see and experience. We must be prepared to keep speaking until we are heard. Our stories have power to change the world around us.

In this compelling and moving book, Duncan reminds us that what really matters is how we respond to other people, and how we recognise that their humanity is just like ours. That is why this book is important and should be widely read.

Barb Spriggs
Australian national human rights award winner, 2017
Senior Australian of the Year, South Australia, 2018
South Australian Most Inspirational Woman of the Year, 2022

Once upon a time …

We are born into a world of stories and storytellers, ready to be shaped and fashioned by the narratives to which we are exposed. The stories we hear and the stories we tell are not only about our lives; they are part of them … We depend on stories as much as we depend on the air we breathe. Air keeps us alive; stories give meaning to our existence.

Art Bochner, 2016[1]

Our world is full of stories. Cultures are created by the weaving of stories – they communicate history and define identities. Stories provide meaning and, in so doing, create context against which we make sense of the events of life. Neurologist and novelist Robert Burton described how our brains are wired for storytelling, experiencing a dopamine-driven boost of pleasure and satisfaction when we sort information into meaningful patterns and explanations – the sublime 'a-ha!' – as he called it.[2] British neuroscientist, Susan Greenfield, has also taught about the meaning-making power of stories. She pointed out that our own life story provides the most important narrative for each of us. Just like all stories, our life story has a beginning, middle and end. It's built around essential plot points – the immutable events that become part of our personal history – tragedy, triumph, suffering and success.[3]

Because we have a story, we can engage with the idea that everyone around us also has a story. This insight is key to our ability to appreciate other people's perspectives and consider what it might be like to walk in their shoes. John Koenig – creative, designer and master of the neologism – captured this idea exquisitely on his website *The Dictionary of Obscure Sorrows* in the made-up word 'sonder', which has taken on a life of its own. Koenig proposed 'sonder' as a noun referring to the realisation that 'each random passer-by is living a life as vivid and complex as your own ... an epic story that continues invisibly around you like an anthill sprawling deep underground'.[4]

What does this mean for us?

Think about encountering people in your daily life. Every one of them has a story. The person before us in line at the checkout; the motorist who cuts us off in traffic; the motorist we cut off in traffic; the people to whom we provide service or care when we are at work; the people we work with. We live in a bustling, chaotic world full of people, who much of the time seem to be charting their own course, interacting with their own sphere of influence, unknown to us and our busy parallel worlds. At other times, people and their stories intersect with our lives and stories – often unexpectedly, sometimes profoundly. What happens in these intersecting moments – how we respond to, engage with, and hold people and their stories – is a litmus test of our compassion and decency as individuals and as a community.

❖ ❖ ❖

I work as a psychiatrist, specialising in the care of older people. I have worked with many older people encountering challenges in their mental health and have been privileged to be invited into their lives to hear their stories. I have also worked with people whose stories have taken challenging plot twists when they have been confronted by the unwanted reality of living with dementia.

While mindful of my responsibility as a psychiatrist to maintain objectivity in clinical reasoning, many aspects of the stories I have encountered have resonated with stories from my own life and family, grounding me in the knowledge that we all walk similar paths through life. My teenage years were affected by my mother's significant depression. My grandmother, mother and aunt all lived – and died – with dementia. My uncle's later years were marked by his struggle with motor neurone disease. Apart from providing a sobering family history, these stories are woven into my worldview, and have informed my work, enriching my service of others.

Life is ephemeral. Wellbeing and relationships are precious. No matter who we are or how we position ourselves we are all much the same – yet the impetus to defend ourselves against the discomforting uncertainty of life can be a powerful influence. The fact is, we are all making our way through life and facing mortality. Our need to live meaningfully – to be heard, understood, and connected with – is a shared experience.

❖ ❖ ❖

Healthcare services around the world are filled with decent people seeking to make a difference and help others. At the same time, in the lumbering machinery of health management, with high demands, resource limitations and cost pressures, it is easy for people to lose their way. This is not a book about the pandemic, but it is necessary to acknowledge that COVID-19 has added new dimensions of complexity to the function and sustainability of health systems, the impact of which will be felt for years to come. Healthcare workers have encountered trauma, stress and discomfort, wrapped up in sweaty PPE (personal protective equipment) and mouth-breathing for hours through their tightly sealed face masks. Communities have experienced uncertainty, disruption and grief.

Deterioration in health services is never straightforward and reflects multiple contributing factors across system and personal domains. What can happen to people who deliver health services – people like me; like my nursing and allied health colleagues, like the health executives accountable for providing services in fiscally limited environments, like the many nonclinical people without whom healthcare would grind to a halt (cleaners, chefs, maintenance staff and administrative officers) – is that they can be worn down and wear out. Motivation can dwindle. Toxicity can creep into organisational cultures. Command, control and compliance can replace compassion and care. Task-based systems, prioritising budgets and service flow over the real-life experience of people seeking help can replace humanity and heart. In these environments, assumptions are easily made, and we stop listening to people's stories.

In 2013, following five years of advocacy and action from families of people affected by the standards in care at Stafford Hospital in the United Kingdom, Robert Francis QC published his landmark report on the Mid Staffordshire NHS (National Health Service) Foundation Trust, which ran the hospital. Between 2005 and 2009, up to 1200 people died needlessly in the hospital. Francis described 'appalling and unnecessary suffering'.[5]

After a gruelling review to unravel the deficiencies in culture and practice occurring in the Trust, Francis provided insight into the complexities of health service failure. He acknowledged the need to consider financial, commissioning and governance issues, but pointed out that it is *people*, rather than *systems*, that 'will ensure that the patient is put first day in and day out'.

He described negative aspects of culture that included a lack of openness to criticism, a lack of consideration for patients, defensiveness, secrecy, an acceptance of low standards, and misplaced assumptions about the judgements and actions of others. He called for 'fundamental change' into a common culture characterised by openness, transparency and candour, with a renewed focus on compassion and caring – modelled by leaders and shared by everyone across the organisation. It is an appropriate vision for all health services.[6]

In 2017, my life changed. I joined a small team, led by Aaron Groves, then South Australian Chief Psychiatrist, to undertake a review of the Oakden Older Persons' Mental Health Service – a specialist aged care service run by the state government of South Australia. The Oakden Campus accommodated sixty-four older people with an enduring mental illness or people living with dementia, who, because of challenging behavioural and psychological symptoms, could not find places of care in the mainstream of South Australia's aged care system.

As our team took a deep dive into the experiences and stories of people living within the facility, their families and the staff who worked with them, we were jointly moved, grieved, traumatised and outraged. Ultimately, we were convinced of the need for pivotal change in how we, as a community, provide care for older people with complex needs and, more broadly, of the need for truly compassionate health and social care for everyone, everywhere.

As we drafted *The Oakden Report*,[7] unaware of the extent to which it would impact Australian health and aged care, we became conscious of the synergy between our findings and those of Robert Francis in his report on the Mid Staffordshire NHS Trust. Oakden was a much smaller service, but for the hundreds of people and their families whose lives were harmed due to its failings, it was every bit as significant.

The Oakden Report caused a furore. It became the centre of a highly public and political scandal, felt across the nation. It became the swansong of the South Australian government after sixteen years in power. It triggered a number of other formal investigations – most notably the Wyatt Review into the Aged Care Quality Agency,[8] the Review of the South Australian Independent Commissioner Against Corruption[9] and the Australian Royal Commission into Aged Care Quality and Safety.[10] What makes the lessons surrounding Oakden so important is recognition that, while it was a *particular* case of failure in system, culture and care, grounded in an antiquated institutional model, it was by no means an *exceptional* case.

After Oakden, stories every bit as traumatic and worse flooded the submissions to the Aged Care Royal Commission. Then, in May 2020, again in Adelaide, the horrific story of Ann Marie Smith, a fifty-four-year-old woman with cerebral palsy, came to light, after her death a month earlier as a consequence of appalling neglect by her disability carer. Once again, there was a national shaking and the calling of a Royal Commission into Violence, Abuse, Neglect and Exploitation of People with Disability.[11]

Let me be clear, while my experiences in relation to Oakden provide an important focus within this book, it is not a book *about* Oakden. Rather, it is a book about *what I have learnt* from Oakden and from other broader experiences and relationships within my life and work. The way treatment was delivered at Oakden was not okay. Compassion, hope and humanity were lost. The reason the stories and thoughts in this book are important is that there are reflections of these losses in many settings. What happens when health systems, and any other service-oriented enterprises, lose focus on the lives and stories of ordinary people is alarming.

❖ ❖ ❖

I have not always worked as a doctor. When I first finished school, I studied classical piano at the Elder Conservatorium in Adelaide with lofty aspirations of a career in the performing arts. A more realistic self-appraisal of my talents coincided with a personal encounter with the Christian faith. Still drawing heavily on music and creativity, I shifted direction and worked in pastoral care, where I met my wife, Lois. I didn't study medicine until I was in my thirties. It has been a gift to me, as a doctor, to remember clearly what it is like to be an 'ordinary' person encountering healthcare, without all the insider knowledge and assumptions that health professionals easily slip into.

I often reflect on an experience in my twenties, shortly after Lois and I were married. As a child, I'd had asthma, but as an adult had largely grown out of any symptoms. One day my hometown of Adelaide was hit by an unprecedented dust storm that created havoc in emergency departments, with many people presenting with severe asthma attacks. I was one of them. I recall my anxiety as I struggled to open my airways and combat the sensation of being unable to breathe.

I will never forget how the doctor on shift spoke with me. He did not use my name, nor his; he talked to me like a teacher condescending to a recalcitrant child.

'Come on, you can blow harder,' he barked, as I huffed and puffed into the spirometer that was testing my breathing capacity. He hurried me along, and I felt belittled and humiliated.

'Typical doctor,' I grumbled, feeling wounded and resentful.

Most important in my recollection of this encounter is how it made me *feel*. This memory informs me as I work with people in my care, hoping that I never make anybody feel the way I did that night.

There are numerous stories of health professionals gaining transformative insight by shifting role from practitioner to patient. Dr Kate Granger was a geriatrician in the NHS in the UK. She was diagnosed with a rare form of cancer and given sixteen months to live at the age of twenty-nine. As a patient she found that many of the staff looking after her did not even introduce themselves. Kate's illness changed her experience of identity. As a doctor who understood the world of healthcare, the contrast between how she *hoped* to be treated and how she *was* treated was significant.

With her husband, Kate commenced the *#hellomynameis* campaign, promoting the simple ritual of health professionals always introducing themselves. She wrote:

> *I firmly believe it is not just about common courtesy, but it runs much deeper. Introductions are about making a human connection between one human being who is suffering and vulnerable, and another human being who wishes to help. They begin therapeutic relationships and can instantly build trust in difficult circumstances.*[12]

Trust and vulnerability are important concepts here. Executive coach, educator and writer Charles Feltman defined trust as 'choosing to risk making something [I like to add '*or someone*'] you value vulnerable to another person's actions'.[13]

As healthcare practitioners we are placed in positions of power. What I do and how I respond to a person in need can have far-reaching impact. Yet we are all also, inevitably, patients ourselves. We should not separate these experiences. One should inform the other. Practitioner; patient; person.

When I place myself or someone I love into the hands of another practitioner or system of care, I am vulnerable. Allowing this insight to penetrate our values can help us reduce the power imbalances that pervade health services. We all hope for people and systems that are *trustworthy* – that will be safe and reliable, that will do good and not harm. These ideas are transferable to many settings and to all forms of government.

❖❖❖

Of course, these issues don't just relate to public scandals like Mid Staffordshire and Oakden. They're part of daily goings-on in health services all over the world.

Not that long ago, my father was admitted to one of South Australia's local hospitals after experiencing dizzy turns. An eighty-seven-year-old retired university professor, he is intelligent, fiercely independent, and entirely in charge of making decisions for himself. I do not dare tell him what to do.

His hospital stay lasted several days. Each day after work I would visit him, and we would have the same conversation:

'Did the doctors come and visit you today, Dad?'

'Well, yes, the consultant came around with his entourage.'

'Did they make any medication changes?'

'I think so. They wrote in the medication chart at the end of the bed.'

'Did they talk to you about that at all?'

'Well, not really. They talked to each other. I couldn't really follow what they were saying.'

'Did they ask for your consent to change your medications?'

'No, they just wrote in the chart.'

'Did you try and speak to them about this?'

'Well, I didn't quite know what to say and there were so many of them.'

My father, who is highly educated, articulate, and used to being in control of his life, found himself in a situation where the power differential between him and the healthcare providers was such that he could not find the confidence to speak up for himself. How would someone with fewer advantages experience this situation? How might this power imbalance be managed by someone for whom English is a second language? Someone from a very different cultural background? Someone with a mental illness? Someone living with homelessness? Someone with changes in cognition?

There are issues here relating to power and control, respect and consent. It is about how the recipients of care are perceived by those providing it. I have worked long enough in healthcare to be confident that my father's experience is representative of many, particularly older, people.

It's not just about older people either. A young woman, in her first pregnancy, shared her story with me. She had been through a difficult relationship break-up and was managing her pregnancy with the heightened anxiety of what life would be like as a single mum. Her pregnancy was complicated by an episode of antepartum bleeding. She attended her local women's health service numerous times, terrified that she might lose her baby.

On one occasion she encountered a male midwifery practitioner whose manner the young woman found disconcerting. As he ushered her into the examination room, she asked:

'Are you able to tell me who my midwife will be today?'
'I will,' he replied.
'I really don't want to be rude,' she went on, 'but is it possible for me to see a female midwife? I'd be much more comfortable with that.'

The midwife did not speak again. He rolled his eyes and ushered the young woman back to the waiting room, signalling for her to sit down. He shut the door on her. Already stressed, she sat in the busy waiting room and cried. Clearly, the midwife did not think about the courage it had taken for the young woman to speak up and express her needs or preferences. He did not consider that there might be a story behind her request to have a woman do the assessment, rather than a man. He did not appear conscious of how the interaction left her disempowered.

Without doubt, a woman in this position needs someone who

gets where she is coming from, who can tune into her story without needing justification or a detailed narrative, and who can work with her to prevent further disempowerment. I have not shared this young woman's story as an argument against male midwives. Rather, the story is a further illustration of how misplaced assumptions and missteps in communication occur every day, affecting all sorts of people.

Why is it so easy for these assumptions to occur? This is by no means a phenomenon exclusive to healthcare. Researchers and thinkers have described perspective-based ways in which people explain both their own and others' behaviours. The common theme is that people routinely misperceive the causes of others' actions, and these misperceptions cause everyday misunderstandings. More concerningly, these assumptions and misperceptions underpin many societal prejudices, inequalities and power differentials.[14]

Back in the 1970s, social psychologists described the idea of the fundamental attribution error (FAE).[15] By definition, FAE is the tendency people have of attributing another person's behaviour to their disposition or personal qualities, rather than to their circumstances or situational factors.

Think of that person who cut you off in traffic – how many of us have had a moment of road rage? We might conclude that the person who did this is rude and lacks a sense of road etiquette. They did it because they're a jerk! But for all we know, they might have been rushing to a hospital or have had some other significant reason for their actions. By contrast, when we are rushing, running late for an important meeting, trying to meet deadlines, it seems quite reasonable to cut someone else off – after all, they're driving like it's Sunday afternoon! Our propensity to tell our own story and overlook someone else's has been demonstrated in research for many years.

Matthew Rice, a consultant with the English health charity The King's Fund, reflected on the idea of unconscious biases impacting our relationships and work lives. He described how our brains are wired to instinctively categorise people based on both visible and invisible criteria – age, gender, race, sexual orientation, religious belief, culture, work discipline and position, and so on. He wrote:

> *Once in a group, we then unconsciously assign that person good and bad characteristics. The evidence around this shows that we are more likely to attribute positive characteristics and therefore have a better relationship with those who appear to be similar to us and share the same values. We all do it, no matter how unbiased we think we are. This bias affects our interaction with colleagues and patients.*[16]

When we perceive people to be different to us, we are more likely to experience discomfort and make negative assumptions about them. Listening to people's stories, openly and sincerely, can help us challenge our own unconscious biases and misattributions. It can help us shift our paradigm to see others as more like ourselves and thus to better understand what it feels like to be inside their experience.

Back in 1989, author and entrepreneur Steven Covey published his seminal text, *The 7 Habits of Highly Effective People*. Covey began his book by exploring a paradigm shift that enabled him to move beyond his attribution error.

He described a journey on the New York subway one calm Sunday morning when a man and his badly behaved children climbed on board and disrupted the whole carriage. The man appeared distracted and oblivious, making Covey irritated. Finally, unable to contain himself, Covey asked the man to control his children. Coming to an awareness of the situation, the man apologised and explained that the family had just come from the hospital where his wife, the children's mother, had died.

Covey's words are telling:

> *Can you imagine what I felt at that moment? My paradigm shifted. Suddenly I saw things differently, and because I saw differently, I thought differently, I felt differently, I behaved differently. My irritation vanished. I didn't have to worry about controlling my attitude or my behavior; my heart was filled with the man's pain.*[17]

Covey's illustration captures the take-home message of the book you are now reading: things change when we connect with other people through their stories.

❖ ❖ ❖

Let's return to the Mid Staffordshire story. Before Robert Francis was commissioned to undertake his review, Julie Bailey, a local woman whose mother had died in the care of Stafford Hospital, persistently fought to have her mother's story heard. She brought together other local people who had similar stories, founded an organisation called Cure the NHS, and drew national attention to the events in the hospital, resulting in the landmark inquiry. She was awarded a CBE for her impact on British healthcare. Julie's story has been retold in a Channel 4 TV drama capturing her tremendous courage and determination.[18]

Similarly, Barb Spriggs, who provided the foreword for this book, persevered against recurrent, systemic resistance in seeking an audience for the story of her husband, Bob, who had Lewy body dementia. He had twice been admitted to the Oakden Older Persons' Mental Health Service. He was frequently restrained. He received injuries that were not recorded but were found incidentally by his family. His physical health deteriorated markedly, and he died. Barb Spriggs continued her mission to tell Bob's story, eventually ending up with a twofold approach: she spoke to the media, and she finally made her way into the office of Jackie Hanson, Chief Executive Officer (CEO) of the Northern Adelaide Local Health Network – the organisation with governance of the Oakden facility.

The power of Barb's story facilitated a deep interpersonal connection and seemed to precipitate a moment of revelation for the CEO, Jackie Hanson. After several years of the budget being the bottom line, Jackie encountered a human story, and realised that she was presiding over a terrible problem. For her, the paradigm shift. Significant here is Barb Spriggs' tenacity in telling Bob's story, and Jackie Hanson's courage to listen and be changed. Like Julie Bailey,

Once upon a time ...

Barb Spriggs was acknowledged for her remarkable and costly journey. At the National Human Rights Awards in 2017, Barb was awarded the Tony Fitzgerald Memorial Community Award for outstanding contribution to advancing human rights in Australia. Then, she was celebrated as the 2018 Senior Australian of the Year for South Australia and, in 2022, as South Australia's Most Inspirational Woman.

❖ ❖ ❖

So, what should you expect from this book? Most importantly, this is a book of stories. It is a book about the power of ordinary people's stories, told with courage, and listened to with curiosity, imagination, and a commitment to learning, bringing about transformative change.

A central narrative emerges from Australia's landmark health and aged care scandal, triggered by the review of the Oakden Older Persons' Mental Health Service. Woven around this are stories from my own life and the lives of people I have met, provided care for, and worked with. I tell these stories to offer a point of reflection, to prompt us to consider what is most important in life and what we might do so that we all live in a more compassionate community.

When sharing stories of those for whom I have provided care, people who lived at Oakden and people from Northgate House and their families, and in several stories regarding healthcare staff, I have changed identities and details to protect privacy. I have sometimes merged details from several cases into new narratives that capture my learning. When writing about my colleagues, I have only revealed identities with explicit consent and deepest respect. When writing about public figures, I have remained consistent with information in the public domain but have provided my perspective on experiences that I lived through and learnt from. I have sought to remain respectful to all the stories captured in these pages while being honest and candid about our shared opportunities to *do* and *be* better.

The stories of people living with dementia, their families and the people and systems providing care for them, create a theme that runs throughout this book. This is important, but this is not only a book about dementia. It is about how healthcare systems and practitioners work; it is about culture and how care is delivered; it is about how people treat each other.

In writing this book, I have been informed by the practice of evocative autoethnography, a reflective research method that connects the personal with the cultural, originated by Art Bochner and Carolyn Ellis.[19] I have also borrowed from former US president Barack Obama's box of tricks. In his 2008 campaign, Obama and his team recognised the power of a practice called the Public Narrative, developed by Marshall Ganz – a unionist turned Harvard University professor. The practice brings together three stories: *the story of me*, *the story of us*, and *the story of now* – the last of which, according to Ganz, is about 'the challenge this community now faces, the choices it must make, and the hope to which we can aspire'. The Public Narrative practice served Obama well, providing a structure for some of his most memorable and captivating calls to vision for the people of the United States.[20]

Given this practice was good enough for Obama, I have used it to scaffold the lessons I felt compelled to put to paper. In the spirit of the truism that everyone has a story, in Part One I reflect on my own story of generations and journeys, setting the scene for how I found myself at Oakden in 2017. In Part Two, we dive into the story of Oakden, and the faltering climb out of failure and scandal. This is a 'story of us' because, while confronting, it is *not* exceptional – the failings of Oakden occur in many places and there is opportunity for learning here for everyone. Important in Part Two are interacting narratives of people and their families, staff who ran or worked in the service and the domains of politics, media and public perception. Part Three is where the music happens, in the redemptive story of a health service for vulnerable people, staffed by broken and wounded people who found their way back to compassionate care by humanising the workforce and reconnecting with people's stories. It is a story about learning a better way to come to work – a change that is precious and, without being nurtured, could be fragile.

As we consider the rich diversity of people we encounter each day, we need to simultaneously hold an appreciation of their individuality and uniqueness, with awareness of our commonality. Every person needs to be welcome; to receive kindness; to tell their story and be listened to; to be understood and treated with respect. We need a compassion revolution in healthcare and across our communities.

We should be aspiring to a better, kinder world for ourselves, for our children and their children. This kind of cultural shift in healthcare and beyond will require belief, time, reflection, vulnerability, and courageous effort. Fundamentally, such change will be built on awareness of our shared humanity – we are all in this together. That is why this is an *everyone* story, and it really matters.

PART 1

Generations and Journeys

1

When I become the other

My older brother's seventh birthday party became a legendary moment in our family history. It gets notable mention even now, many decades later. It was the 1970s and we lived in a gracious, between-the-wars, verandaed red-brick bungalow in one of Adelaide's leafy eastern suburbs. There were three of us; my older brother, Andrew, me, and my younger brother, Robert – a baby just a few months old.

We had a wide grassy front lawn, which on this day was set out with a catering table holding party food and big, red-striped buckets of Kentucky Fried Chicken. At the party were about fifteen rambunctious boys, all having consumed too many lollies and too much red cordial (who knows what my mother was thinking?), who were then given swords and shields crafted out of hard cardboard and sprayed metallic silver by my father.

It wasn't long before our front lawn degenerated into a warzone for the whole, fairly gentrified, community to see. At some point, someone decided that swords and shields weren't enough and yelled, 'Hey, let's get the birthday boy with Kentucky Fried!' Within seconds, drumsticks, bread rolls, lollies and whatever food was left over burst over the scene like a finger-lickin' rain cloud.

I was five years old and very different in temperament from my brother and his friends, being much more interested in quiet and crafty pursuits than winning wars. I was keenly aware of this difference and completely terrified by the debacle. I retreated to the veranda, where my much-loved maternal grandmother pulled me onto her lap, into safety and solace, quietly whispering, 'I think we might stay right away from those boys at the moment.' I recall both my parents leaping to action in their efforts to contain the ruckus.

It is widely known that grandparents and grandchildren can have a special bond. Unfettered by the responsibilities that colour the dynamic between parents and children, there is the possibility that grandparents and their grandchildren engage with fewer expectations of compliance, cooperation or achievement, such that they can simply *be* with each other. I had that comfortable kind of knowing-without-words relationship with my grandmother. When I step back into the memory of that moment, I can almost convince myself that I can smell her, feel her softness.

Connection and comfort were more influential in my relationship with my grandmother than her cognition or capacity. To start with, I had little awareness of her early stages of memory loss or how this limited the things she might be able to do. I never noticed that she did not babysit us by herself, but only with my grandfather present. For a while, I was blissfully ignorant of the conversations adults in my family had about what appeared to be happening to her.

When I was older, I learnt my grandmother's story from my mother. She had been the eldest of three daughters born into a middle-class South Australian family at the end of the nineteenth century. Her family owned a successful sports store in the city and a rambling stone house near the Adelaide foothills. My grandmother and her sisters attended St Peter's Collegiate Girls' School, where they were provided quality education by Anglican nuns at a time when many young women's expectations remained constrained by the need to marry and raise the next generation.

The context of my grandmother's story, of which my mother made sure I was aware, was that her family had freely migrated from England to build a new life in South Australia, bringing their sensibilities with them. By contrast, my father's family came from convict stock transported to New South Wales early in the nineteenth century. My grandmother epitomised the idea of a more genteel vintage era. My father's Scottish convict heritage provided a contrasting, but gratifying, point of identification.

At the same time, my grandmother's story reflected courage and quiet determination. After finishing school, she defied her father's directive that she should abstain from seeking further education and employment and should prepare herself for marriage.

'No daughter of mine needs to work,' her father said.

My mother proudly recounted how my grandmother stood up to him and declared her intention to train as a teacher, which she did, becoming the first woman in our family to complete tertiary education. She worked as a Montessori preschool teacher, which, remarkably, made her something of a radical at the time. She went on to marry and raise her family, working alongside my grandfather as they moved around Australia with his employment as a bank manager.

Her self-determination as a young woman became another defining plot point in our family story. Her daughters, granddaughters and great-granddaughters have been inspired to take progressively further ground in each generation, as women convinced of their absolute equality with men, with the right to live and work without limitations. I am very grateful to have this knowledge of my grandmother's story and strength. It makes me immeasurably proud of her.

My mother also told me the story of how, when we moved from Australia to live in Oxford in the UK for a time, my grandmother, for whom memory was becoming increasingly imprecise, experienced distress. Confused by the loss of the grandchildren she loved and unable to hold on to my grandfather's reassurances that we would come back from the UK, she would repeatedly ask to go to our house in Adelaide, saying, 'I have to look after the boys.' We did come back, and I reconnected with my grandmother. By that time, the threads of adult commentary regarding the changes occurring for her had coalesced.

'Nan has senile dementia,' I was told. I didn't fully understand what this meant but got the sense that it redefined her identity. It placed her in a category of *different* and, unintentionally, in the ignorance of such declamatory nomenclature – *senile dementia* – it threatened her value. It was my first exposure to the powerful impact of ageism and the marginalisation of people with dementia, expressed through the inherent attitude and language of the 'othering' of older people.

❖ ❖ ❖

Othering is a foundational concept, relevant to all the lessons gained through the stories expressed across the pages of this book. Othering accounts for dynamic differentials in power between dominant 'in' groups and disempowered 'out' groups – categorised against all sorts of defining characteristics.[1] The concept of othering digs deeper into the attribution errors and misaligned paradigms considered in this book's introduction.

Unbeknown to me at the time, I was already familiar with the impact of being othered, having daily experienced the social rigours of a primary schoolyard, where differences deemed unacceptable by peers were translated into repeated moments of bullying.

I was a particularly unathletic child. Had my life depended on my ability to throw a ball or lob a rock, I would not have made it beyond the age of eight. When I was in grade three, the PE teacher, Mr Brown, unceremoniously gave up on me. We had to throw a tennis ball over a soccer goal. After a few unsuccessful, dyspraxic attempts, he grabbed the ball from me and chucked it on my behalf so that we could all finish up and go home. I was the child who was always last at the selection of sports teams, with the two captains arguing over why they shouldn't have to tolerate the liability of picking me.

'You have him.'

'No, *you* have him!'

My mother would console me after school by trying to convince me of age-old wisdom regarding sticks, stones, bones and names. Even then I knew this was rubbish.

'Of course names can hurt me,' I said to myself as I buried the psychological trauma under a defensive stance towards my peers, pretending that what happened didn't make me feel less than human.

I tell this story not to garner pity but because I know I'm not the only person to have experienced the excruciating shame of such moments. While living through my early induction to being 'othered', I had no concept that this kind of experience could continue to occur throughout a person's lifespan, nor that it was the ubiquitous experience of all manner of individuals and communities. I was yet to understand that this process underpinned the plague of social and political disempowerment and inequality around lines of race, gender, age, sexuality, faith, politics and culture that has characterised human history.

Simone de Beauvoir, the great twentieth century French feminist philosopher, wrote about this phenomenon, providing a foundation for her arguments regarding the experience of women and older people:

> No group ever sets itself up as the One without at once setting up the Other over against itself. If three travellers chance to occupy the same compartment, that is enough to make vaguely hostile 'others' out of all the rest of the passengers on the train. In small-town eyes, all persons not belonging to the village are 'strangers' and suspect; to the native of a country all who inhabit other countries are 'foreigners'.[2]

Othering involves identifying similarities and differences to determine who belongs to social groups. These groups don't have equal power, and this has implications for superiority and inferiority, privileges and punishments, gains and losses.[3] Groups that hold more advantages – wealth, strength, ability, age, gender, social influence – get to decide who does and does not belong. The consequence is the dehumanisation of those who are 'other'.[4]

In his book *Modernity and Ambivalence*, sociologist Zygmunt Bauman poetically captured these group identities and power relationships. He wrote:

> Abnormality is the other of the norm,
> deviation the other of law-abiding,

illness the other of health,
barbarity the other of civilisation,
animal the other of the human,
woman the other of man,
stranger the other of the native,
enemy the other of friend,
'them' the other of 'us',
insanity the other of reason.[5]

I think we can add to Bauman's list:

Patient is the other of practitioner,

old is the other of young.

We could go on – there are many others.

In Western society we are youth-obsessed. Our deep aversion to ageing is counterintuitive, given one of the things we ultimately have no control over is the passage of time. No amount of Botox will change the inevitable reality that we all grow old. We will all, eventually, die. It is likely that in the years before death we will encounter increased frailty, illness and the need for help and care from other human beings. Understandably, most of us prefer to not think about this. Most younger people see older people as very different from themselves – like they're a different species. They can't conceptualise what it will be like to actually become old.

At its worst, the public prejudice regarding ageing is characterised by imagery of impending doom. The popular media metaphor of 'the silver tsunami' has been used to depict the overwhelming of social and economic resources, like some pending epic natural disaster. Search Google images and you'll easily find the classic satirical cartoon by Canadian artist Graeme Mackay, which points out the absurdity of this metaphor. It depicts a terrified group of younger ('normal') adults on a beach about to be obliterated by a giant wave of deathly grey zombie-like older people, complete with walking frames, newspapers and knitting.[6]

I am not dismissing the necessity of health economics and planning. Nor am I denying the importance of the promotion of preventative initiatives that will support an increase in the numbers of people achieving healthy ageing without the burden of chronic disease. The problem with the language and imagery here is that it effectively dehumanises older people, making them appear a resented burden to be carried by the young. This is not helpful. It impedes conversations that accurately and respectfully represent universal issues of ageing.

Modifying the young–old dichotomy, to some degree, is the population of people who are 'middle-aged' – somewhere between youth and old age, aware of differences between themselves and their emerging adult children, while supporting the increasing care needs of their now ageing parents. Moments of realisation will flash into the consciousness of this population as they realise that, little by little, they are becoming less the other of the old and more the other of the young.

A few years ago, I completed research in which I interviewed psychiatrists about their experiences of working with older people who were approaching the end of life. Several themes emerged from these conversations. The psychiatrists in the study talked about how, early in their careers, they saw their older patients as very different to themselves – they perceived these people as 'other'. The psychiatrists found it easy to remain personally distant from the problems these people brought with them. As time passed and the psychiatrists began to encounter issues arising from their own ageing, they had to come to terms with the diminishing gap between themselves and their patients. This uncomfortably compelled the psychiatrists to contemplate their own ageing and mortality. 'Them' started to shift closer to 'us'. The falsehood of othering became increasingly apparent.[7]

Many older people refer to the experience of 'feeling invisible'. They find themselves taken less seriously in the workplace or overlooked in social settings.[8] This conveys a compelling state of 'otherness', which is magnified for people with other points of difference – such as dementia.

Tom Kitwood was a psychologist, researcher and writer about person-centred dementia care, which places the person needing and receiving care at the centre of the care system – not the process of care, nor the facility or staff. In person-centred care, the person is understood, and their preferences and choices appreciated and respected. Yet, as Kitwood pointed out in his influential book, *Dementia Reconsidered: The person comes first*, people with dementia often experience being invisible and being characterised as 'less than human'. When arguing for dignified, compassionate, person-centred models of care, Kitwood asserted: 'There is to be no us–them divide.'[9]

For many cultures and throughout history, intergenerational households have been a normal way of life. Elders have been revered as members of the community and there has been reliance on younger generations to provide care through incorporating older people into family and community life. Contemporary Western lifestyles tend not to look like this. Although few Western older people want to live in intergenerational households – for fear that it might limit their independence – there is food for thought in intergenerational models. Research demonstrates the powerful, heart-warming, bi-directional benefits in understanding, relationships and wellbeing of programmes promoting intergenerational learning between children and older people.[10] If you need to be convinced, just watch a few minutes of the hugely popular TV show *Old People's Home for 4 Year Olds* – either the UK or Australian versions – it's inspiring and you'll easily be hooked.[11-12] What better way to undercut the othering of older people and address the perpetuation of ageism than to build respectful, curious, learning relationships between children and older 'storytellers'?

❖ ❖ ❖

The last time I saw my grandmother was during a holiday visit back to Adelaide after my family had moved to Bathurst in New South Wales. Because we lived far away, I had not witnessed her transition from independence to dependence. It was the late 1970s and she was living in a nursing home. She could no longer walk and had lost most of her language, saying only a few syllables. I was too young to form a reliable understanding of the quality of care she received, but my recollection is of her lying in bed in a room with several other people, in an environment that appeared much like a hospital. It smelled clinical. My memory has none of the ease of a comfortable homelike space.

I recall my grandmother picking at the flowers on the plastic curtain around her bed. With my medically informed hindsight, I wonder if she was delirious. There was awkward conversation about her not being able to recognise who we were. My mother told us it was okay to wait outside but I felt a strong sense of connection that remained for me, beyond words. This was my grandmother – still soft, lovely, and comforting – and I wanted to be with her.

My grandmother died later that year. Perhaps it was a sign of the times that my mother, who was devoted to both her parents, did not travel from Bathurst to Adelaide to attend the funeral. It was too far, too expensive and too complicated, and so instead she stayed home, visited by her friends while she listened to a recording of the choir of King's College Cambridge singing hymns that both she and my grandmother loved.

As children, with the future stretching like eternity before us, my brothers and I recovered from the news of our grandmother's death without being aware of the impact on our mother. It was only as an adult, considering this period in retrospect, that I questioned why my mother would not have returned to her family to grieve with them, or why my father would not have thought it essential for her to go and for him to go with her. Was it too hard? Was it something about dying with dementia that made it less critical to honour the moment, the loss, and the life? Had the underlying state of otherness changed the landscape?

I remember my parents describing the relief of it being over. It was my first exposure to the conflicted feelings that families often encounter because of dementia – relief and regret, grief and guilt, all jumbled up together. I know my mother struggled with enduring disappointment that circumstances had not afforded her a better opportunity to grieve the loss of her mother or honour her story.

My grandmother's story holds several threads at once. For the women in our family who came after her, she modelled independence and mould-breaking, going against the norms of her time. She was a wife and mother, who laboured with love and commitment. For me, she was a much-loved grandmother who provided comfortable warmth and relational connection simply because of who she was.

As the first point at which dementia intersected with my story, my grandmother introduced me to the potent influence of ageism and the marginalisation of people with dementia. Her story coalesces with my own childhood experiences of being othered, with its emphasising of difference in ways that steal power and threaten our shared humanity. If it were not for the convergence of my grandmother's story with my own, perhaps I would not have been ready for later lessons that would shape my direction in life. Through my grandmother I began to appreciate the change and loss resulting from dementia, alongside the need to hold firmly to an understanding of the person and their story, recognising that their humanity and value remain, throughout and beyond the limitations of age and illness.

2

I'll like you for always

It's sometimes suggested that the therapist becomes a therapist to solve their own problems. There is, undoubtedly, interplay between the insight that comes from one's own experiences and the motivation and ability to help others. In my case, I have no doubt that I became an old age psychiatrist, at least in part, because of living through my mother's illness. There's a fine line between sorting out the issues such an experience leaves you with and placing yourself in a situation where you can make a difference for others and the community. We are all embedded in the generational stories wrapped around us. These contribute to the way we form and function within our worldviews.

My mother was the youngest of three children. The eldest, Jeanne, was self-assured and in control. Raymond was in the middle, good-looking and suave, always able to talk his way through a situation. Younger by several years was my mother, Elizabeth Clare, diminutive and shy. 'Little Elizabeth' was how the more confident family members referred to her, suggesting a more delicate disposition and lesser resilience than her older siblings. She struggled to throw off this uncomfortable moniker, even after establishing her own family, all the while seeming to suspect that it may have held some inconvenient truth for her.

My mother was born in Jamestown, a country town in South Australia, after the Union Bank stationed her father there. Because of his work, the family moved multiple times. My mother was enrolled in a succession of schools across South Australia and Victoria, limiting her ability to establish friendships that might have grounded her early years. Despite this, she maintained a playfulness and loved being outdoors, albeit often spending time alone.

One of her closest companions was her cousin Rodney, who was similar in age. She later delighted in telling stories of the naughty-but-innocent antics they got up to when he visited from Adelaide. She would tell of how the two of them would climb a tree at the back of the bank building that was also my mother's home and throw berries over the churchyard next door. Particularly rewarding was her story of sneaking in behind the toilet, which in an Australian country town in the 1940s was outside and involved removable buckets and a plank of wood with a hole in it. Reaching through a trapdoor at the back, my mother and Rodney would push a stick through and poke her imperious sister's bottom.

My mother finished her schooling at The Friends' School in Hobart, where she became a prefect. She spoke fondly of her days at the school and was aware of the apparent contradiction that 'Little Elizabeth' became a school prefect despite her shy, apologetic nature. Her story encouraged me that introverts need not be relegated to the role of follower.

In Hobart, my mother's family once again lived upstairs above the Union Bank. The bank was directly adjacent to a popular hotel where the Indian cricket team stayed during their 1948 tour, in the days when Don Bradman captained the Australian team. My mother gleefully told us the story of how the bank provided a kitchen and dining space large enough for the visiting cricket team to cook and host a dinner of a scorching hot curry. My mother's family was in attendance, my grandfather – a devoted cricket fan – chuffed by his celebrity guests.

After Hobart, the family moved back to Adelaide, a homecoming to the place where both my grandparents had been born. My grandfather took up his final post: a prestigious appointment as manager of the Adelaide ANZ Bank, in Edmund Wright House, a stately Victorian building on King William Street in central Adelaide. It was here that he proudly claimed the title of Bradman's bank manager. Meanwhile, the family moved into a comfortable bungalow in the suburbs.

My mother turned her attention to nursing training, which she completed through the Queen Victoria Hospital for women and children, going on to train as a midwife. She achieved the second-highest graduation score in her year, behind her best friend Cicely Bungey – another of the more confident and assertive circle of friends and family with which my mother surrounded herself lifelong. It was Cicely and her husband Colin who years later set my mother up on a blind date with their mutual friend John McKellar, hoping that, finally, these two thirty-somethings would find someone with whom to share their lives. The matchmaking was successful, and Cicely remained a faithful, beloved friend to my mother throughout the remainder of her life.

My mother's most joyful stories were from her years as a nurse and midwife, particularly in the late 1950s when she travelled to London, with Cicely and another friend, Jan Adams, to live and work as young Australian women abroad.

My mother worked at the Great Ormond Street Hospital for children. She would tell us stories of her time there and show us pictures of herself wearing her pointed nurses' cap. Alongside her time living in Oxford, with my father on sabbatical and my brother Andrew and me as small children, these were times of delightful adventure for my mother. Listening to her stories evoked a romantic vision that elevated the UK far beyond the ordinariness of central New South Wales.

❖ ❖ ❖

Reflecting on my family's move from Adelaide to Bathurst in the mid-1970s, I am struck by how other people – particularly the men in her life – took control of my mother's destiny. My father was a committed academic, eagerly looking for an opportunity for advancement and feeling stymied in his post at the South Australian Institute of

Technology. A chance to undertake a Head of Department position arose at the Mitchell College of Advanced Education in Bathurst, which was redeveloped in the late 1980s as Charles Sturt University. It would have been reasonable for this decision to be explored by my father and mother together. Indicative of the remarkable tenacity of 1970s chauvinism, my father and grandfather – my mother's father – asked my mother to step outside of the sitting room while they discussed the issue. They summoned her back in for my grandfather to say, 'Elizabeth, I think it best that John takes this opportunity and you and the family move to Bathurst.'

Why on earth she did not object, demand some opportunity to make her voice heard, to rail against a decision made on her behalf, without her engagement, I never understood. What is clear is that she was about to enter the most problematic years of her life. No amount of effort to reconcile the favourable outcomes the move may have had for other members of the family could negate the impact on my mother. The rationalisation, 'If it had not been for moving to Bathurst', became part of our family story through most of our years there and beyond, yet it failed to resonate as a positive note in my mother's narrative.

My mother did not fully recover from the grief associated with the loss of place, family and connection resulting from her dislocation to Bathurst. She had found a home in one of Adelaide's verdant and comfortable suburbs, close to her parents. It was a gracious home, well-positioned near quality schools and shopping precincts. After an early life spent moving from town to town, she had felt established and settled, with the hope of a positive future – including her anticipation of returning to work as a mothercraft nurse after the birth of her third son, Robert.

She arrived in Bathurst in early winter. It was bitterly cold, with a fog that lifted at 11:30 am only to return at 4 pm. She was confronted by repeatedly sick offspring, cramped rental living quarters and an increasingly absent, work-addicted husband. She desperately missed her parents and the comforts of home. Her mother was continuing to progress through dementia, and my mother wrestled with the guilt of not being able to provide support. When purchasing a house in Bathurst – a sign that this would be an enduring move – the 1950s brick veneer held none of the charms of her lost home in Adelaide, despite a spectacular view across a local valley.

My mother became depressed. It was the late 1970s and early 1980s in country NSW. Even now, literacy regarding mental health and illness is often limited and stigmatised. Back then there was no local mental health service, no visiting specialists, and local GPs delivered all healthcare. It was before the era of readily available or tolerable antidepressant treatments and psychological therapies. Through my contemporary lens as a psychiatrist, I see the symptoms of severe depression, with biological features that called for treatment and psychological contributors reflecting grief, loss, and disconnection. Instead, my mother struggled with her distress untreated, apparently poorly understood by her doctor, appearing increasingly alien to her children, and a source of frustration to my father. She spent many hours lying on her bed, and I can still hear the desperate, heaving, habitual crying that became a persistent soundtrack to that period of our lives. There is nothing that redeems this memory for me.

❖ ❖ ❖

There is a high prevalence of depression in dementia.[1] The extent to which my mother's depression was a harbinger of the clouds that were to wrap themselves incrementally around her memory and function is unclear. For some people, symptoms of depression may be the first signs of neurocognitive change.[2] Where dementia is not a factor, depression can be followed by recovery, and by a life lived with greater insight and empathy. In my mother's case, her distress abated, but she was never the same again.

The discovery of a lump in her breast further complicated my mother's journey through depression. Once again, the limitations of treatment in 1980s country NSW meant that she had a limited choice of surgeons. She underwent a bilateral mastectomy and lymph node clearance. Following surgery, she made multiple trips to Sydney, where she would stay in a hostel for cancer patients for six weeks at a time, receiving radiotherapy. The treatment was gruelling, irradiating a large portion of her upper body, with side effects that included burning, pain, and severe fatigue.

My father's mother came to stay with us while my mother was away, to keep the family running. She did so with military precision and a sustained emotional distance. I yearned for my mother and felt continuously uncomfortable with my paternal grandmother's presence.

My mother later talked about her experience with cancer treatment. Particularly notable was her description of a review appointment with her surgeon – an upright, formal, older man. He had her take off her top, bra and prosthesis. Gazing down at her disfigured chest, he smiled with satisfaction and said, 'What a lovely scar.' My mother, acquiescent, said nothing, but she later confided to me that she wished she had swiped back at him, 'I preferred what was there before, thank you.' It was her nature to think of the retort after the event. What a disappointment some medical practitioners cannot see the person behind the scar.

❖ ❖ ❖

My mother was in her fifties when she began to show the telltale signs of neurocognitive change. We all noticed her trouble remembering things, the word-finding difficulty, the loss of already limited confidence, but nobody commented. We quietly knew the history established by my grandmother's illness but hoped that if no one acknowledged it, we wouldn't have to deal with the reality.

Matters became more problematic. People noticed and expressed well-meaning concern. By this time, I was living in Adelaide, studying music at university. During a holiday back home, I saw my much-loved piano teacher, and she cautiously inquired, 'How is your mother? Is her memory okay? People are worried about her.'

Then my mother left the lettuce crisper in the laundry basket on the back lawn. And one day, she parked the car, got out and walked away, leaving the door wide open. There was no way that she nor we, as her family, could continue to ignore the unsettling truth that awaited acknowledgement on our family agenda.

Rounds of medical assessments commenced. Initially, my mother's mini-mental state examination score – an internationally recognised, albeit blunt, screening tool for dementia providing a score out of thirty – was in the low twenties. Doctors kindly euphemised, describing her as having 'mild cognitive impairment'. This was technically true, based on the testing, providing an opportunity for us to hope for the best while the doctors took time to break the bad news gradually. In 1992, just as she turned sixty, my mother was formally diagnosed with dementia, likely Alzheimer's disease. By then, she had been symptomatic for several years.

When my mother was diagnosed, I had recently married. Lois and I were living in a cheap, tiny but trendy one-bedder in Adelaide's foothills. I was in my twenties, with high hopes for the future. Even with my mother's diagnosis, as a young adult, the concept of mortality and the challenges of ageing felt personally foreign. It is likely protective that the dawning realisation of mortality usually comes to people in mid-life, as otherness shifts direction.

Early on, my mother retained capacity. She understood what her diagnosis meant and was aware – at least to some degree – of the anticipated progress of her illness, having witnessed her mother's experience. Her diagnosis was distressing because of what it meant for her and because of the familial ramifications. She struggled with guilt and misguided responsibility. I remember the day she tearfully lamented, 'What if I have given this to my boys?' We all comforted her, reminding her that this was not her fault and that it was more complicated than family history. While a portent of future concerns, the reassurance giving enabled us to suppress the issue of genetics, leaving this to trouble us later.

❖ ❖ ❖

Up to ninety per cent of people with dementia encounter some degree of behavioural and psychological symptoms.[3] These include a wide range of experiences such as mood changes, agitation, anxiety, changes in perception and beliefs not based in reality, through to aggressive behaviour towards self or others. Symptoms also vary through degrees of severity from mild to extreme.

The terminology 'behavioural and psychological symptoms of dementia' can be controversial.[4] It may be that this very clinical language fails to capture either the experience of people living with dementia or that these symptoms reflect limitations in communicating personal needs or processing environmental stimuli. Pain, hunger, thirst and toileting needs are all common causes of agitation for a person with dementia, often because that person is not able to tell others how they are feeling.

It may be that somebody with dementia appears paranoid, developing a belief, for example, that people are entering their home overnight to steal or damage property. For some, this can develop into complex delusional beliefs, such as people living in the ceiling or being able to move through doors or windows without unlocking them. We can find the genesis of these delusions in the process of altered memory and sense-making. I have worked with people with dementia whose narrative of intruders 'stealing' from them can be explained by the simple misplacing of their possessions.

Themes of trauma from earlier in life can resurface through these symptoms.[5] This can be deeply troubling for people with dementia, and for their families and carers, who struggle to manage the impact on the quality of life and the capacity of services to provide care. These symptoms do not last forever and usually abate with the further progression of the illness. Nevertheless, the period during which behavioural and psychological symptoms become a predominant concern is generally the most challenging time for the families of people with dementia.

In my mother's case, her symptoms remained moderate for several years and she was able to continue living at home. Nevertheless, it was a disquieting period for us as a family. She experienced depression and significant anxiety. As her physical function deteriorated and her gait became more faltering, her fear increased. She became overwhelmed by the noise and busyness of public places. As a result, my parents did not visit shops or go to large gatherings together. She experienced episodes of agitation and was treated with haloperidol, a first-generation antipsychotic. With medical hindsight, I suspect she did not need this pharmacological intervention, which made her gain weight, become more slowed and sedated, and further impaired her gait.

She found it increasingly difficult to identify people she had known and loved. It was incredibly painful when I ceased to be distinguished as a son and was recognised only as a familiar person. Most distressing was when my mother could no longer recognise her own reflection. Clinically, this is a delusion of misidentification – or, more casually, the 'mirror sign' – and is reasonably common in people with Alzheimer's disease.[6] When confronted with her reflection in a mirror or any reflective surface, such as the oven door, she would become highly distressed, perceiving the image as an unknown and hostile intruder. One day, after my parents had moved back to Adelaide from Bathurst, she angrily raised her fists to attack her own image in our hallway mirror.

'That dreadful woman,' she hissed at her unrecognised self.

We took the mirror down. My father diligently covered the reflective surfaces in their home, seeking to avoid the trauma of these moments. The simmering vehemence that erupted in my mother at these times, seemed to capture the grief and anger she experienced over the progressive loss of self and identity – feelings she was unable to voice in any other way.

❖ ❖ ❖

The marriage vows that pledge devotion and care through ill-health take on deep meaning in a chronic, degenerative illness such as dementia. At a time in life when people hope they will be able to enjoy an ambling pace in retirement, the partners of those with dementia find themselves enduring an unexpected and gruelling marathon.

They are often increasingly alone, with the person with whom they have spent their life becoming progressively less accessible yet more demanding.

The role of carer did not sit naturally with my father. He was a driven university professor whose discipline was inorganic chemistry – definitely not a 'soft' science. His early life history, education, career and personal choices all reflected someone smart and focused – but less inclined to prioritise interpersonal relationships. Throughout my childhood, I witnessed the deficit my mother quietly tolerated in my father's ability to cue into her emotional needs, concerned as he was about his work and the machinations of office politics.

It is to his great credit that my father intentionally changed his life and dedicated himself entirely to his role as my mother's advocate and carer. Having spent his adult life pursuing career advantage, he retired early from a senior position at Charles Sturt University. After they moved back to Adelaide to be close to my young family, he built his retirement around my mother's changing needs. He went through a transformation because of this experience that resulted in a more connected version of himself.

It was not an easy role, caring for my mother. For a man who was quick to solve technical problems, a challenge such as helping her get in and out of the car when she had lost the ability to sequence and perform simple motor tasks was vexing. My father would bark orders in frustration, only for my mother to become more confused and flustered. I would watch in anguish and advocate for a gentler approach while trying to remain respectful of my father's primary role. He understood, intellectually, that my mother was not being deliberately obstructive, but the emotional rigours involved in getting through the many practical tasks of the day proved a constant source of tension.

'I keep telling her what to do,' he would say frustratedly. To which I would reply, 'You know that she can't remember or follow instructions. It's not her, it's the illness.'

This conversation remained on a loop for a long time – an experience that is widespread for partners and families of people with dementia. They are doing their best to provide care to their loved one while under a continual pressure that inhibits their ability to access the reflection and patience required to remain even-tempered. This is a challenge that must be navigated and overcome, but we should not perceive it as the fault of those struggling to provide care.

My mother had worsening difficulties with incontinence. She would routinely wet the bed overnight, and my father struggled to cope with the use of continence aids. Falls increased and, because of the weight gain from the use of antipsychotics, it became more difficult to help her up from the floor. Fortunately, I lived around the corner, and my father would ring me most times to come and assist in getting her up – although sometimes he risked injury and did it himself.

After battling on valiantly, matters finally became too much for my father. He called me one day when my mother had been faecally incontinent in the living room and then fallen into the mess. My father was distressed and unable to get her up.

'You cannot do this anymore,' I said to him, 'it's more than you can manage. You've worked really hard, but this is not good for you and it's not good for Mum.'

Overwhelmed and exhausted, my father agreed for my mother to go into urgent respite within twenty-four hours. Apart from day visits, she never returned home, and transitioned into permanent care in a residential aged care facility.

The decision to place a loved family member into residential aged care is often heart wrenching for families and fraught with guilt. Australia's aged care system has suffered from patchy levels of quality across providers, as well as adverse media reporting and poor public relations. In recent years, the sector has been impacted by the Oakden-triggered Royal Commission, followed promptly by the traumatising impact of the pandemic and austere lockdowns.[7] Many older people and their families navigating the transition into aged care have lost confidence. Yet the reality is that the tasks required to provide care for people with many of the morbidities of ageing – most notably dementia – often become more than families can deliver themselves at home and it becomes a necessity to trust others with these responsibilities.

For my father, despite his reluctance to relinquish his role as my mother's primary carer, it proved a tremendous relief to be free of the physical tasks involved in attending to her proliferating needs. Instead of daily struggling with these tasks, he was able to realign his attention towards their relationship. I saw more tenderness from my father in those final years than I had witnessed throughout our family life. He visited my mother almost every day. We often had to encourage him to take days off and make time for himself. He advocated for my mother to be understood and honoured by the staff in the facility. He became the archetypal 'agitating relative' regarding aspects of care he considered below standard. He witnessed the limitations of staffing ratios in the facility and determined that he would support my mother through a daily mealtime, ensuring that she received adequate nutrition, rather than risking meals being hastily delivered, and then left on an over-way. Most notably, my father talked to my mother, held her hand, hugged her, kissed her – continuing to do so beyond her grasp on language or any ability to reciprocate.

Having a keen, strategic and visionary mind, and a broad capacity for organisational leadership, my father took on dementia as a cause with the assurance of someone who understood how it impacted life. He joined the Board of Directors for the Alzheimer's Association in our state, quickly ascending to the position of Chair – a position he held for more than a decade. He represented South Australia nationally and for several terms held the position of national Deputy Chair. It was a flourishing time for the Alzheimer's Association in South Australia, with many new initiatives, positive inroads into the community, and organisational growth. It allowed my father to sublimate some of the persistent grief of my mother's slow decline into something positive; it fuelled a fighting drive to create purposeful change. As a result, he was awarded a Medal of the Order of Australia and named as Senior Australian for South Australia in 2001 for his work as an advocate, leader and carer.

❖❖❖

The journey towards my mother's death was conflicted and painful for all of us. In the early years of dementia, she was diagnosed comorbidly with precancerous bowel changes. We decided against treatment. In the last two years of her life she experienced recurrent anaemia, indicative of chronic, life-sapping bleeding in her gastrointestinal tract. By then, I was in medical school, armed with sufficient knowledge to think I understood issues around treatment choices. My father, as a primary but exhausted advocate, tried to make ethical decisions on my mother's behalf and struggled with his own need to continue to care. My mother's GP vacillated between consideration of the broader context of her prognosis and quality of life, and concern over the classic medical conviction of needing to treat, as well as anxiety over how it might be perceived to *not* treat.

Because of this rolling uncertainty on how to proceed, my mother received numerous blood transfusions. She repeatedly came back from the brink of death, to once again have my father battling with her care providers over the day-to-day issues of support with feeding, continence and repositioning in her 'princess' chair – a deeply curved, vinyl-covered-foam, chair-on-wheels, lying back in a semi-reclined position. I am uncertain how much quality she found in the life that was extended for her during this period by those of us doing our best to decide. I cannot, nevertheless, say that she did not find meaning, or that she was oblivious to the love or connection we sought to provide her. Dementia, and our own confusion, settled like a thick blanket over our sense-making of her experience.

I closely identify with families who find themselves in a quandary as surrogate decision-makers. Aching grief juxtaposed with guilt over self-perceived betrayal jostles with deep weariness and a desire for the journey to be over. Knowing how and when to let go is a decision which, even if pre-empted in earlier discussions and advance care directives, remains emotionally distressing. Is this the time? How do we stop clinging to life and allow death to no longer be a feared enemy? I suspect that underpinning this uncertainty is our shared human struggle with mortality. What if this were me? Even in the face of personal losses caused by dementia, would I be ready to go? How can I make this choice for another?

Irrespective of our ambivalence and hesitation, there is a time for everything. There came a time when it was evident that the focus of my mother's care must, without question, be on the end of life. Dying is life's final milestone and dying well is one of the most outstanding collaborations between people and those who provide care. My mother had lost her ability to swallow safely and developed an infection that made consideration of the further treatment of anaemia irrelevant. A new challenge emerged as the alleviation of pain, breathlessness and distress began to appear beyond the capacity of the care team in the residential facility.

Older people have been described as 'the disadvantaged dying'.[8] At times 'comfort care' may be used as a euphemism for not assessing or responding to terminal distress. In my mother's case, the impotence we encountered in advocating for management of her terminal symptoms in residential care was the last source of angst – most potently experienced by my father. We were greatly relieved when my mother was transferred to a local hospice, where the relief of her symptoms was like a soothing salve to us all. The nursing staff in the hospice responded to us with simple kindness, respect and flexibility that created a safe harbour.

With her pain eased and breath coming only intermittently, my mother slipped through the veil that makes the momentary difference between life and death. My father sat at her bedside, holding her hand. I was not present at the time and arrived after my wife. We hugged and cried. Touching my mother's hand for the last time, I felt the warmth already dissipating from the physical body she no longer inhabited.

The death of someone deeply loved is a strange experience. The aching absence of the person contrasts with their continuing presence through memories that incorporate multiple senses and moments in time but remain delicate and require deliberate intention to bring into focus. I remember my mother as she lived with dementia. More profoundly, I remember the gentle, compassionate and sensitive woman, who thought of others and considered their feelings; who devoted herself to her children; who told stories of her childhood and days nursing and travelling.

During my mother's illness and at the time of her death, I found comfort in *Love You Forever*, a children's story written by Robert Munsch. The story describes the unwavering love of a mother for her son, following him throughout his life, singing him a simple song of commitment each evening. The story poignantly closes with this mother growing old and no longer being able to hold her son or reach the end of the song. Instead, her son holds her and repeats the song to her, before going home to hold and sing to his own child – the next generation. As I reflect on the inextricable intersection between my mother's story and my own, I am confident that there are no better words than Munsch's:

> I'll love you forever,
> I'll like you for always;
> As long as I'm living,
> My mother you'll be.

3

Jeans and genes

I did not know my Uncle Raymond well. He married many years earlier than my mother did, his children adults before I was born. I remember little of my older cousins, with a vague recollection of my cousin Warwick on my parents' front lawn, briefly visiting before he left the country to pursue a career in equine medicine in the United States, never to return. Uncle Ray's wife, Aunt Jean, was an only child. My parents told me this by way of explanation when I complained that she was 'scary'. Uncle Ray was successful in the corporate sector, and I recall their lovely home, designed with Jean's excellent taste and preferred accoutrements. As a child, I felt intimidated by 'the rich Baylys'.

As a reminder that wealth provides no guarantee against misfortune and illness, Uncle Ray was diagnosed with motor neurone disease at sixty. I was still a teenager and my mother yet to become symptomatic. Our families were not close. Separated by both relationship and distance (we were in the central west of New South Wales and the Baylys were scattered across the globe), I did not see Uncle Ray during his illness. Instead, my aunt relayed updates to my mother. They would discuss the developments with sadness and concern, and then my mother would report to our family.

At the time, the reality of Uncle Ray's illness seemed abstract to me. Some years later, with my mother increasingly unwell, I better comprehended the suffering couched in stories of Uncle Ray's progressive decline. First, he had to stop working and then he needed increasing help at home; this was followed by the skulking theft of walking, speaking, swallowing and breathing. Uncle Ray died, leaving Jean bereft and once more alone.

Scientists have identified more than twenty-five genes that contribute to the onset of motor neurone disease. The most commonly associated gene is found on chromosome 9. Humans have twenty-three pairs of chromosomes (including our sex chromosomes X and Y) and these carry the genes that give us every biological feature we have. This particular motor neurone gene (called C9orf72) is also associated with frontotemporal dementia – a type of dementia that affects the front part of the brain responsible for making decisions and managing behaviour.[1] People with this gene might present with motor neurone disease, dementia, or a combination of both. Other genes passed on in families can trigger the disease, or cases might be 'sporadic' – occurring in an individual, independent of their family history, when a new gene mutation occurs. There is still more to be understood regarding the genetics and interrelationships of these illnesses. But having a family tree with multiple occurrences of potentially related illnesses can cause considerable anxiety.

❖ ❖ ❖

My other Aunt Jeanne, my mother's sister, was a precious person in my life. Her three daughters were, to my brothers and me, like sisters who lived nine hours away in Melbourne. We remain close to this day. School holidays, spent with our cousins at their beach house on the Mornington Peninsula, forged idyllic memories for us all. We still look back at these as halcyon times, overlooking the regular teases, tiffs and tears.

We called Jeanne 'Aunty Jell', short for jellybeans, which might suggest she was sweet and colourful. But as much as I came to love Aunty Jell, she was anything but sweet. Smart, focused, intensely choleric, Aunty Jell remained formidable throughout her adult years, just as she had been through my mother's childhood. This was counterbalanced by her husband, Uncle Jack – a gentle, forgiving, pipe-puffing man who would end most conversations with a reconciliatory sigh and 'Oh well, never mind'.

My mother and Aunty Jell loved each other dearly and, at times, fought bitterly, even as adults. My mother forever felt she was in Aunty Jell's shadow, overlooked and in the way. Aunty Jell always considered herself within her rights, as the eldest by many years, to be the boss. Despite their disagreements, they would reliably restore their relationship and they shared an abiding connection. My mother's death was a moment of deep grief for Aunty Jell, notwithstanding the relief that the suffering had ended.

Aunty Jell was in her eighties when she was diagnosed with dementia, likely Alzheimer's disease. Living in Melbourne, she was able to access care through an eminent professor and one of Australia's leading dementia researchers and clinicians. My cousins – a general practitioner, speech therapist (married to a leading geriatrician) and a nurse – attended appointments to support Aunty Jell, who was, by this stage, widowed. On reviewing the family history, complete with our grandmother's illness, my mother's younger-onset and our uncle's motor neurone disease, the professor furrowed his brow. Providing some consolation to my cousins, he stated, 'Well, if you had to choose, I'd say your branch of the family tree would be the preferable option.' Small solace to celebrate the later onset of dementia.

Aunty Jell's progress through dementia was less dramatic than my mother's. Increased frailty accompanied her changing cognition and function. She transitioned with only minor difficulty into a quality residential aged care facility, where she was much loved by the staff. Recreating her life as a social worker, the team invited her to sit in the nurses' station and gave her papers to manage, providing a sense of connection to people and purpose.

❖❖❖

As a doctor, many families ask me if dementia is heritable. I strongly identify with the anxiety these family members encounter while summoning the courage to untangle this Gordian knot. I seek to respond with compassion and truthfulness – recognising that these are what I would need myself. The pain and anxiety experienced by these family members must be acknowledged, without seeing it as in any way degrading the dignity of the people with dementia, for whom they grieve.

I explain that some specific types of dementia have known genetic relationships, but there are relatively few families where this is very clearly the case. More commonly, family history is a factor that increases risk, but it is not the sole factor or a fait accompli. Multiple factors contribute to the risk of dementia.

Dementia is in the top ten causes of death worldwide and is the second most common cause of death in high-income countries.[2] It is the leading cause of death for women in Australia.[3] Investment in research is important to shed new light on the causes of dementia and to provide hope of prevention, delay, and a different pathway through the disease. There is a need for drug research to continue, in search of medications that will both prevent and reverse the toxic proteins that accumulate in the brain and cause dementia. At the same time, research regarding modifiable risk factors offers hope of healthier ageing – undoubtedly worth people with high-risk family histories exploring. The fact is: healthy ageing is for everyone – including people living with dementia.

For some families, an aberrant gene can become a troublesome feature in their story. In more recent times as a psychiatrist, I provided care for a man called Henry, who had younger-onset dementia – which by definition means the onset of illness before the age of sixty-five. Henry was diagnosed with dementia at fifty, but his wife, Angela, said that he had trouble with his memory from his late forties. The family was devastated but not surprised – both his father and his older sister had been diagnosed around the same age, with similar symptoms.

Given the family history and young age of onset, Henry and Angela decided that he should go through genetic testing, worried about the implications for their children, teenagers at the time. Henry was found to have two copies of a gene called APOE e4 on chromosome 19. The gene affects the brain cells' ability to process fats and is known to increase the risk of Alzheimer's disease significantly – especially in people who have inherited two copies of the gene – one from each parent.[4]

Henry's diagnosis changed his family's life. They cared for him at home until it was no longer physically possible, when he went into an aged care facility. It was awkward and uncomfortable for Henry, as a fifty-three-year-old man, being admitted to a facility where other residents were much older than him, many in their eighties. It was before the introduction of the Australian National Disability Insurance Scheme, which applies to people with younger-onset dementia – but even with this, we still have a long way to go to ensure that younger people with dementia have access to quality care suitable to their stage of life.

Fortunately, the facility was a good one, with hopeful, flexible leadership – ready to bend rules to make things work. What was important to Angela – who provided the resilient strength that held the family together – was that she could stay involved as much as she wanted as Henry's primary carer, and his wife. She could be as hands-on as she wanted but could let others step in when she needed to take a break. Still raising three teenage children, she needed to go home at the end of the day and be Mum.

Henry's father's and sister's illnesses followed a similar course – five years from diagnosis to death. But Henry had complicated symptoms. He developed psychosis – a change in mental state where he became paranoid and started having frightening, torturous hallucinations – seeing images of strange creatures attacking him. He became distressed and agitated, unable to differentiate between what was real and what wasn't. It was terrifying for him and everyone caring for him. His fear, distress and disorientation were expressed through self-protective but violent behaviours.

Henry's symptoms needed treatment with an antipsychotic – but he had side effects to most medications, limiting options. The specialist palliative-care team helped manage Henry's intractable restlessness. It was an extraordinarily difficult time, and after weeks of struggle, Angela yearned for Henry's suffering to be over.

Then, all of a sudden, things changed. Whether it was getting the mix of medications right, or a marker of how his illness was progressing, Henry settled. It was like a cool and calming mist descended on his room, holding a moment of sacred quiet.

His family sat by his bedside. Angela held his hand. After all the suffering and confusion, Henry roused from sleep, appearing briefly to come to almost-coherence.

'Hey love,' Angela whispered tenderly, 'how are you?' A pause and a hint of a smile.

'I'm good,' said Henry before slipping back to sleep.

The following day he died. He was fifty-four.

After he had died, Angela gave consent for post-mortem studies that confirmed his diagnosis of dementia with features of both Alzheimer's and Lewy body diseases. This finding explained his symptoms and why he didn't tolerate some medications – a typical feature of Lewy body disease. The family grieved and healed – but were left with the lingering legacy of what to do about the genes. Two generations profoundly impacted by illness. What about the third generation and beyond?

❖❖❖

Another family with whom I have worked had many members across generations with either frontotemporal dementia or motor neurone disease – or both. The family participated in research contributing to understanding of the C9orf72 gene that can cause both diseases – important for science but deeply troubling for the family.[5]

I met Kathy during the Oakden review. She was one of the long-term residents at the Oakden Older Persons' Mental Health Service, where she endured significant deprivation. After the Oakden Report, she moved to the fledgling replacement service at Northgate House, where she became one of the best teachers on how to deliver better care.

Kathy had watched her father live with dementia in his sixties. Kathy presented with the onset of symptoms in her early forties. Just when she expected to be raising her children, enjoying her family, advancing her career, travelling, and living her way, Kathy experienced a progressive syndrome of being 'locked in' and unable to communicate. She became increasingly dependent on others. Because she was so young, she did not carry the burden of physical frailty or medical issues that many older people do at the onset of dementia. Instead, she was highly active and easily bored. She was placed in institutional care at Oakden because there was no other facility or funding available at the time able to respond to her needs.

The heart of Kathy's family was her mother, Dawn. She had nursed her husband and supported his sisters through dementia. She stepped in to raise Kathy's children. She tenaciously advocated for Kathy and warred against systems of care that were inadequate. She sat on committees and boards. She wrote letters. She faithfully visited and cared for Kathy year after year. Spared the distress of having the gene herself, and fortified by uncompromising strength of character, she remained the matriarchal glue that held her family together. All the time, she navigated her own ageing, managing the anxiety raised by the question, 'What happens for Kathy when I am gone?'

Nearly twenty years after Kathy's first presentation, her sister, who had chosen not to have genetic testing, presented with an unusual episode of severe psychosis, where she developed a range of detailed delusional beliefs – ideas not based in reality. She was admitted to hospital for assessment and care. The illness caused by the C9orf72 gene can initially present as psychosis before noticeable memory changes emerge. Unfortunately, results from Kathy's sister's memory tests were consistent with the start of dementia and the family was faced, again, with the demand to adapt.

It is challenging to consider how any of us might respond to the question, 'Should I be tested for this gene, or not?' Even more troubling are the questions that come tumbling out after the first. 'If I have the gene, what should I do?' 'If I don't have the test, will I just live with anxiety – or denial?' 'Should I have children?' 'Should I use IVF and test the embryos?' 'I've already had children – what if I've passed this on to them?' 'If I have the gene, can I prevent the illness?' 'Who do I. tell?' 'Can I get health insurance?' 'How do I plan my future career and finances?' 'What do I do with my life?' 'Do I want to live with this?' 'How will knowing change things?'

Questions such as these are why health services recommend that individuals and families in similar situations sit down with a counsellor, to work through what undertaking the process of genetic testing means and what they may need to consider if confronted by an unwanted result.[6] The decision to seek genetic testing is no small one; ethical implications regarding who might access the results and how they might be used require careful consideration. The involvement of several clinicians from various disciplines – medical specialists, GP, psychologist and social worker – is recommended for good reason. Time and nuanced conversations are helpful. The ability to remediate genetics antenatally offers hope for future generations. Still, genetic studies may result in grief for individuals confronted by frightening news, even if other risk factors are modifiable.

❖ ❖ ❖

After my mother's death, given my father's scientific predilection, we consented for tissue from my mother's brain to go to the Australian brain bank for diagnostic clarification and research. Pathology testing confirmed that my mother had died with Alzheimer's disease, providing us with an opportunity to undertake genetic testing from my mother's sample. The fact that we did not know what we might discover was disconcerting and raised all the obvious questions. Part way through the process, I found myself gripped with anxiety and wondering what I would do if we got bad news. Would I get myself tested?

There are limits to genetic testing, based on current knowledge and available technology. At the first panel of tests, shortly after my mother's death, none of the genes known to cause Alzheimer's disease were present. Twelve years later, the genetics service contacted our family again, offering a further panel of tests based on new knowledge and technology. Once again, no known genes were identified, including those associated with the connection to my uncle's motor neurone disease.

There was comfort for my brothers and me in these results. Nevertheless, family history is what it is. I understand the emotions experienced by families living with dementia. It is simply not possible to divorce oneself from the stories of earlier generations.

We all hope for blissful, trouble-free lives. But disruptive and painful things happen to entirely decent people. The challenges of the future are unknown and myriad. We need to live well now despite this.

In his revered work *Man's Search for Meaning*, Viennese psychiatrist Viktor Frankl articulated his treatise on the relationship between life, suffering and death. Frankl earned his right to speak about existential issues through his journey of survival, interned in Theresienstadt, Auschwitz and Dachau concentration camps during World War II. He wrote:

> *If there is a meaning in life at all, then there must be a meaning in suffering. Suffering is an ineradicable part of life, even as fate and death. Without suffering and death, human life cannot be complete.*

Frankl asserted that a person 'may retain his human dignity even in a concentration camp'. He described the responsibility to choose one's attitude in any circumstance as 'the last of the human freedoms'.[7]

Science and technology have given us the ability to modify genetics for future generations, but for those of us already walking the earth our family history and genetics are non-modifiable risk factors. This fuels the questions and anxieties that people and their families bring with them into doctors' rooms, hospitals and aged care settings every day. One of the reasons we tend to make older people and those with dementia *other* than ourselves, is because it helps us keep these questions at bay. But there are risk factors that we *can* do something about, and it's up to us how we relate to these. What's more, as we are reminded by Frankl's hard-won wisdom: our attitude to the uncertainties of life is within our sphere of influence. Not easy – but life changing.

4

Changing lanes

My work as a psychiatrist with older people is a part of a continuing vocational journey. The idea of *vocation* is about more than identifying a preferred career pathway. Vocation brings together the threads of life – personal, professional, relational, spiritual – living and working in a way that provides an expression of who we are. In a probing set of essays, author and educator, Parker J. Palmer, drew on the Quaker wisdom encapsulated in the statement 'Let your life speak' and asked the question, 'Is the life I am living the same as the life that wants to live in me?'[1] He referred to a process of 'becoming myself', drawing from a classic poem by American poet May Sarton, that describes 'trying on other people's faces'.[2] This implies ongoing reinvention, movement, and testing things out – a continued 'arriving', rather than a concrete 'having arrived'.

The stories of my grandmother, mother, uncle and aunt provide important context for my process of 'becoming'. So, too, do the stories of my personal Christian faith, challenging experiences within the church, and my mid-thirties lane-change into medicine. These set the scene for how I came to be at Oakden in 2017 and help make sense of what I would learn when I got there.

I made a personal commitment to a Christian faith while I was at university, studying music, then teaching. An open-heartedness toward God had been percolating for several years, inspired by my mother's return to faith during my teenage years. As a younger child

I had attended a local church with my family – my mother sincerely committed; my father in attendance; myself with childlike receptivity but limited understanding.

My family stopped going to church after the local minister had a relationship with one of the church elders, and their respective spouses fell into each other's arms in consolation. The community considered it scandalous. My parents could not reconcile the way things were with the way they 'should' have been, and we did not attend again until my mother found a new spiritual home at the local Anglican cathedral. I then witnessed her life settle after years of carrying a sense of loss. Her spiritual restoration caused me to reflect on the calling to my own pilgrim's journey – albeit a reflection coloured by issues of adolescent angst and confusion.

I took up residence in St Ann's College at the University of Adelaide and, while sorting through the mayhem of opportunities offered in college life, encountered fellow pilgrims, also spiritually searching. Together we embarked on a journey of faith that was sincere and transformative.

My life of faith has not been without challenges, frustrations, or battles with doubt and disappointment. In fact, the tough times have brought greater benefit to me than the transcendent 'mountaintop' experiences. Nevertheless, the life-affirming about-face I experienced answered the inner moral and spiritual dissonance with which I struggled and has informed my life ever since.

I became part of a church community where I met Lois, and our relationship grew in tandem with our shared yearning after vocation. We had our children and raised them on a mat laid out on the church floor. Our life was busy, devoted, and hopeful. Memories of my grandmother, while precious, dimmed. My mother's illness grew as a shadow swelling over the horizon.

After several years of lay leadership within the youth and music ministry teams, I took up full-time employment on the pastoral staff. I gained valuable skills in working with people, communicating, public speaking and leading. In later times, when working in healthcare, I would often find myself leaning back into what I learnt from the years in ministry. I found myself more seasoned in the art of therapeutic conversations than many of my peers, reflecting my years in pastoral care.

There were difficult lessons as well. Churches, like all human organisations, are at risk of drifting away from important values and behaviours. We are all familiar with the public failings that have plagued some churches – and various other organisations – following the uncovering of horrendous stories from survivors of childhood sexual abuse. Reports have emerged in the media of the leadership and moral lapses of numerous celebrity church leaders. Financial and sexual indiscretions have damaged reputations, disrupted communities, and destroyed families. There have been accounts of church cultures discoloured by bullying from controlling leaders who have succumbed to hubris – above rules and conventions, without accountability to other people, and having lost sight of their roles as servants rather than commanders.[3]

Starting as a slowly simmering change in culture and practice, I encountered the damaging influence of a deviation from authentic, servant-leadership, and witnessed the impact of hierarchical power differences and the infiltration of othering in attitude and language in the church that was both my workplace and my community. It became an environment in which speaking up about problems was perceived as disloyal and became personally risky.

My intention is not to defame any church, nor to deter anyone from exploring the fundamental tenets of Christianity. My point is this: when I later encountered the dehumanised culture associated with the Oakden Older Persons' Mental Health Service, where the system had lost connection with the person and their story, and where people didn't speak up because of fear of either punitive action or uninterested inaction, it was familiar to me because of what I had learnt from hubris-infused leadership culture in the setting of my church. Deterioration in culture can occur anywhere – in churches, health services or any other enterprises. I am convinced that the way back is through reconnecting with simplicity, humility, and compassion; maintaining respect for everyone and openness to their story; welcoming well-intentioned differences of opinion – creating cultures where it's safe to call things out when needed.

Lois and I found ourselves unable to safely express concerns about our observations and experiences, and so, feeling there was no alternative, we left the church we had considered home. For a time, we joined the ranks of the walking wounded of the church. Fortunately, in the intervening years, the church we left has found its way back to a more positive place, as have we.

❖❖❖

My journey out from working for the church and into an entirely new career in medicine and psychiatry occurred in tandem. Retrospectively, the segue into medicine saved me: had there not been a new opportunity, the trauma of lost relationships and work within the church may have been a far more destructive burden.

My first inkling of emerging problems within our church leadership culture coincided with the surfacing of quiet discontent surrounding my work and direction. My tasks and roles in ministry in the church seemed to have lost their challenge. I started to wonder about my growth and vocation. How would I sustain the work I was doing? Who am I, anyway, and how is my work a reflection of me? I felt a restless stirring for reinvention – the disquiet of vocational discovery.

Early in this journey of changing lanes, I bumped into a family friend, Jeff, an airforce officer who was studying in the Flinders University graduate entry medical program. We talked at length about his experience of deciding to study medicine. He spoke with warmth and fluency about his experience and, unknown to him, as he talked, I felt his words igniting deep confidence in me. It was as if I was listening to my own story – one that I was yet to live. I didn't talk to anyone about it, not even Lois. I hid the moment away for a further eighteen months, while continuing to feel increasingly stuck in the status quo.

For many years I had glibly lamented that I had not studied medicine when I left school. But I was not that serious – when I was eighteen, all I was interested in doing was playing the piano, with no thought of practical goals. I was academically successful, but the idea of medicine was synonymous with success in the sciences, and I had an internal script that told me I was an arts student, lacking aptitude for chemistry, physics, and biology – considered the medical student's essential foundations. It took me years to challenge this presumption.

And then, one ordinary Sunday afternoon in July 2001, an extraordinary event occurred – like coming upon an unexpected signpost. I still don't have a rational explanation for it.

It was a typical weekend. We sat down with a cup of tea – Lois to read the book she had on the go, me to read the Sunday paper. I opened the paper to a photograph and story about three first-year students in the Flinders University graduate entry medical program. With everything that had been ruminating in me for the previous eighteen months, it was a lightbulb moment. One of the students in the photograph was a music graduate in her mid-thirties. Here was evidence, in my hands, that people like me got to reinvent themselves and head off to university in their thirties to study medicine.

Without pausing for thought, I turned to Lois, holding the paper up to show her.

'Look here!' I ecstatically declared. 'This is the course I'm going to do!'

Lois and I may have been on the journey of change together, but we were not at the same junction. Conceptually, she saw us as people working in Christian ministry, and the thought of stepping outside of that identity remained foreign to her – even though she was on the verge of commencing her doctorate, part of her journey into the world of university research and teaching.

'Don't be ridiculous!' she retorted. 'We're in the ministry. You're not doing that to me and ruining my life.'

Not the embracing response for which I might have hoped.

'Well, I'm going to apply and see what happens,' I snapped back.

'You do that,' she said, firmly believing that the obstacles would quickly appear and push the idea out of my head.

Lois turned back to her book, *Think Big*, the personal account of Ben Carson, MD. Carson overcame a highly disadvantaged early life to become one of America's most celebrated paediatric neurosurgeons. Lois commenced reading at the very next paragraph:

> *Knowledge makes people special. An example that comes to my mind is W. Duncan ('Fred') McLeary, our sons' paediatrician. Fred trained to be a teacher and taught in the elementary schools. In his thirties he decided he would rather be a physician, so he applied to and was accepted by a medical school.*
>
> *Did Duncan waste his training as a teacher? Some might think so. As a parent, however, I am convinced that because of his teacherly love for children, Fred has transferred that skill and information over to his work as a paediatrician. And we, the parents and patients, gain from his vast knowledge.*[4]

For a moment, Lois debated with herself. 'Do I tell him what I just read?'

The parallels were bizarre – including the fact that, as a child, my parents had called me by the nickname 'Fred'. The sceptic might view this as a ridiculous coincidence, but the passage arrested our attention. Was it possible that God was trying to speak to us through these events? Were we crazy to be thinking this way?

I told Lois about my earlier conversation with Jeff, and what had been growing in my thoughts for many months. She remained cautious, and we agreed that we would carefully test the water – preparing for whatever might eventuate.

The process involved several steps. First, I found the student from the story in the Sunday newspaper, who, as it happened, only lived a few blocks from us. She gave me some great advice and provided material to help me prepare for the GAMSAT – the graduate medical school admissions test. At first glance I almost lost hope, overwhelmed by language and content that seemed alien to me. But it provided me with a starting point to bridge the gap between my previous knowledge and what I needed for the future.

Trusting that this was a vocational step in the right direction, I put time into my preparation for the entrance exam, discovering as I did, that I was able to perform well in the science curriculum I had thought was off-limits for me. On the day I walked into the exam hall, filled with anxious applicants, most of them a decade younger than me, the room was tense with nervous energy.

'I'm only giving this one shot,' I said to myself. 'It's this time, or never.' Fortunately, I performed well and made it to interview, and then to the first round of admission offers.

It felt surreal to enter medical school with a class that included people from around the world, younger and older than me, with diverse backgrounds, from health sciences through law, education, and the arts. An exponential period of growth was ahead. At the same time, Lois embarked on her doctorate. Our young family – Elspeth and Erin in primary school and our youngest daughter, Edie, just six months old – adapted to a new normal, with busy parents and almost no money. We lived frugally, worked hard, and were constantly challenged. Life was good.

❖ ❖ ❖

Medical school behind me, I began my internship at the Lyell McEwin Hospital, in Adelaide's northern suburbs, among some of the most disadvantaged communities in Australia. Up against inequalities of resourcing within state health services and with significant social determinants of health impacting the population – unemployment, generational poverty, reduced health literacy – the hospital managed to retain a pioneering spirit. The new interns were well supported, and we forged positive relationships through long hours and new challenges. It is fair to say that internship turns the medical student into a doctor.

In my second rotation as an intern I worked in Howard House, the acute inpatient unit of the older persons' mental health service. The rotation was a turning point. Like stepping into my vocation, it felt like coming home.

Howard House was situated away from the Lyell McEwin Hospital, on site at the Oakden Campus, next door to the long-stay service that was to be the focus of the Oakden Report years later. The building was old and tired, but the staff were kind, hardworking and delivered quality care with commitment. The unit was later moved to a new building at the Lyell McEwin Hospital, connecting it with the main part of the hospital and separating it from the decline occurring in the remaining services.

As a naïve intern, my exposure to the rest of the Oakden Campus was limited to a few short calls, to relieve the resident medical officer. My recollection of these forays into the extended care units is of spaces populated with very disabled people seeming to wander without a clear purpose, or reclining in princess chairs – in hindsight, likely restrained. (The term princess chair is deeply paradoxical – suggesting a means of providing greater comfort and elevating the incumbent person to a higher status; yet, in this context, it was a way of restricting movement and freedom, resulting in less frequent interaction with care staff.) I filled in medication charts and reviewed residents who'd had falls and then quickly left, feeling awkward within the milieu. At that time, I was not able to piece together my sense of discomfort with a coherent awareness of there being systemic problems within the unit. It took several years to understand what can go wrong in health services.

My trips into Oakden aside, I loved my work in Howard House. I loved the patients. I loved the consultants and staff who worked there. I loved rubbing up against humanity, threaded through with complex problems, and the requirement to consider more than the presenting complaint. Some days I would help a person navigate a seemingly insurmountable problem. Other times I would be excited to see someone recover and go home to resume their life.

I would be amused by the comedic goings-on of the ward. I remember, in colourful detail, an incident involving two women with advanced dementia, both called Joan. One Joan emerged from the bathroom holding a feculent gift in cupped hands, gleefully received by the other Joan, who started spreading it around on walls and furniture at lightspeed. I have never seen such a flurry of activity from nursing staff as they leapt into action to contain the mess. Shamefully, I bid a hasty retreat.

The idea that I might have found my clinical homeland edged into my thoughts – a homeland populated with the ultimate underdogs: older people with mental illness or complex behavioural symptoms resulting from dementia – people that many other clinicians, and the community, seemed to find confronting and therefore aversive. It seemed to me that these people might be the ultimate 'others' of the health system. I had found what felt like a noble cause, resonant with meaning and purpose.

Having passed through the internship rite of passage, I qualified with full medical registration and continued as a resident medical officer at the Lyell McEwin Hospital. My first position was in community mental health, working afternoons and evenings in the emergency department and doing rapid response community visits to people in crisis. The service covered the far northern suburbs of Adelaide. Limited opportunity took its toll on these communities. I started to think that the great nation of Australia might not be so great: such confronting disadvantage within kilometres of leafy-green affluence. The impact of drug and alcohol use was palpable in the emergency department and in my numerous visits to provide reviews of young men expressing suicidal thoughts after being incarcerated at the Elizabeth Police Station.

I moved on to a rotation with the palliative-care team. Here I was immersed in the stories and experiences of people and their families as they navigated the final significant developmental challenge in life – dying. Working at the edge of humanity attracted a particular type of person and cultivated a culture of care that stood in stark contrast to the fluorescently lit hustle of the acute hospital services.

These experiences convinced me that my future was in psychiatry, focusing on older people as they manoeuvre through later life development, including the inevitable task of approaching the end of life. The most language-rich of medical disciplines, concerned as it is with story and meaning, psychiatry played to my strengths within the humanities and connected with my values and motivations. Focused and organised, I progressed on schedule, commencing specialty training in old age psychiatry in my fourth year.

Although the service had moved to its new accommodation at the Lyell McEwin Hospital, I returned to work with the same team I had worked with in Howard House several years earlier as an intern. I revisited the Oakden Campus, covering further short calls when needed. With more experience under my belt, I had increasing awareness of the many problems associated with the service, from the degree of resourcing through to the deficient culture.

There were no jobs available in old age psychiatry when I graduated. I took a job working in adult community psychiatry in the eastern suburbs of Adelaide. I learnt much about how services and systems work and began to have a vision for how a team might look, built around positive relationships predicated on trust and honest communication. After eighteen months, a job in old age psychiatry was advertised, and I commenced working at the Queen Elizabeth Hospital in Adelaide's western suburbs.

And so, I had effectively changed lanes, while still travelling the same vocational road.

In his book *Visions of Vocation*, theologian Steven Garber repeatedly challenged the reader to ask the question: 'Knowing what I know, having heard what I've heard, having read what I've read, what am I going to do?'[5] We live in a world where there is suffering, pain and injustice. How can we know what we know and not despair?

I experienced deep disappointment after encountering an example of deteriorating culture and integrity in the church. It would have been easy to throw out faith because of failure. Working in Adelaide's disadvantaged northern suburbs, I struggled to reconcile the inequalities present in my own community – privilege and poverty;

health and hardship; side-by-side. And this is before considering equity more globally. Moral distress might render us disabled – or worse, cynically hardened to the needs around us.

Garber posed the question: 'How can we know the world and still love it?'

Believing that my life has purpose, and that I have an opportunity to make a difference in the world, gives me the hope I need to keep living vocationally.

5

Meet the teachers

Lectures and textbooks are often a necessary part of learning, but the most valuable lessons in my early years as a doctor came from people who shared parts of their lives and stories with me. With retrospective critical reflection, these 'teachers' helped me grapple with what it means to provide care in a complex world. I will share just some of these stories, and what they taught me as a foundation for further lessons when I arrived at Oakden in 2017.

I recall a lesson from my first week working as the resident medical officer with the Northern Crisis Intervention Service. I attended an urgent assessment of a young man whose partner had called in, upset.

'He says he's the devil,' she'd reported on the phone. 'He's not normal, and we're really scared.'

It wasn't clear whether he'd been taking amphetamines or some other substance or whether he had a pre-existing psychotic illness. There were small children in the house and, concerned to avert an escalation in risk, a social worker and I quickly headed out to assess him at his home, several suburbs north of the hospital, just as day eased into dusk.

We arrived at the young man's home in tandem with the police. Police attendance was common practice to manage the security risks around such a situation. I can only imagine how it must feel to be confronted at home by clinicians from mental health services, accompanied by police.

The local community, by contrast, appeared to enjoy the show. The street was populated with low-lying semi-detached single-storey bungalows built from economic grey concrete blocks. This was the most affordable government housing of the sixties and seventies, with little maintenance through decades of hard living. Broken chain-link fences and dusty front yards completed the streetscape. Sensing excitement, several neighbours gathered with deckchairs and stubbies to watch the show, set against a blazing sunset.

We knocked on the door. The police stood back. A young woman, puffy-eyed and perspiring, greeted us.

'He's out the back,' she said, ushering us inside. 'I'll ask him to come through.'

We cautiously entered to find a young family in pandemonium. There was litter everywhere. The woman invited me to sit on a dirty lounge, among dried leftover pizza. I remained standing, awkwardly, in the centre of the room. There were three small children, all under five – one naked from the waist down, roaming through the litter, followed by two slender, sniffing dogs of indeterminate breed. My colleague, who had many years' experience, took the lead.

The young man and subject of our visit came in, unhappy and embarrassed about us being in his home. Beneath close-cropped blond hair and multiple facial piercings, he looked gawkily young, even adolescent. He was not psychotic. He admitted to smoking plenty of cannabis but insisted that he did not use amphetamines.

There were many challenges for this young family. We were struck more by their unpreparedness for the demands of relationship and children than by any immediate risk of psychosis. There had been an altercation and claims had been made about the devil, but to have medically pathologised this would have been to miss the real work needed through support, education, persistence and patience.

My social worker colleague, who was known for his equanimity, understood the family systems issues at play. He led the couple through an impromptu work of conflict resolution, before recommending some connections to local non-government family support services.

There was no trip to the hospital. The police went back to their patrol, and the neighbours considered their options for alternative evening entertainment.

Through this experience, and other early visits, I gained respect for the perspicacity of my social worker colleague. I learnt that there are families everywhere who have conflicts and deficits and yet love each other. Perhaps most importantly, I learnt that it is easy to pass judgement without knowing the whole story.

Sometime later, I attended a call-out with another clinician. A suburban landlord had reported concern about a woman who had not paid rent in weeks. We attended the woman's home. She was from Korea and spoke very little English, so we took an interpreter with us.

The woman appeared cautious, but finally allowed us inside. Her power had been cut off. It was winter, and she had no heating, no way to cook food, and no working refrigerator. She was spending most of her time in her bedroom, which she had lined with aluminium foil. She had built a fortress around her bed with cans of food and bottles of water, like a cave she would crawl into. She wore a helmet fashioned from aluminium foil, like a crude primary-school science project.

Through the interpreter, we deciphered a convoluted story about alien invaders and her need to protect herself from their intrusion into her thoughts. She was unquestionably psychotic, unable to manage her life at home sustainably. She presented with likely schizophrenia. I made an order under the *Mental Health Act*, and she was transported to the hospital for assessment and treatment.

It was one of the first times I had deprived someone of their autonomy by placing them under such an order. In this case, I was confident that it was the right thing to do. It was the pathway to ensuring she'd be in a safe, warm place where she could have a shower and a warm meal, with the hope of engaging in treatment that would ease her symptoms.

In many subsequent encounters, the decision to interfere with a person's autonomy would be less black and white. I would wrestle with the balance between the criteria stipulated in the Mental Health Act, and the person's right to manage their own life – even if that looked very different to what might seem best to me.

❖ ❖ ❖

Time and training moved on, and my work became more focused on older people. I became thoroughly familiar with the 'three D's' of older persons' mental health – depression, dementia and delirium – learning that these are seldom straightforward and are underpinned by the uniqueness of each person's story and circumstance. But the stories and problems that older people brought to our services were not limited to textbook alliterations, they offered diverse lessons in the complexities of life and care.

I met Esmelda, a sixty-seven-year-old woman, occasionally still selling her skills as a clairvoyant. She was eccentric and flamboyant – and provided a cautionary tale for anyone thinking that 'older' people don't use hard drugs. She was admitted to hospital several times with episodes of drug-induced psychosis – disorganised, with bizarre delusional beliefs, following binges on amphetamines.

With the community mental health team, I visited the home of Macklin, a small, jockey-sized Irish man in his seventies, close to losing his tenancy because of his hoarding. The council had given notice that his home was a hazard to public health and a mandated clean-up was imminent. His house was barely habitable. He slept in a chair and ate cold tinned food, unable to get to his bed or the stove – both buried under papers, purchases, bits and pieces.

I visited Diedre, a seventy-year-old woman with severe obsessive-compulsive disorder (OCD) – an anxiety disorder characterised by intrusive, anxiety-provoking thoughts (obsessions) and driven patterns of behaviour used to alleviate anxiety (compulsions). OCD can range from mild to severe – at which point suffering and disablement can be extreme. Diedre's life was completely held to ransom by OCD.

When I arrived at Diedre's house with a colleague, the curtains were drawn, and it seemed deathly quiet. Diedre answered the door and I reeled at the acrid smell of bleach – it was like entering a fastidiously cleaned laboratory.

Meet the teachers

Diedre was a slender woman, with shoulder-length greying hair. She looked exhausted. Her hands and forearms were pastily pale from hours spent ritualistically washing and cleaning. Fear of impending doom lurched constantly at her. She couldn't stave off the conviction that the only way to prevent cataclysmic disaster was more cleaning.

I offered Diedre access to our team psychologist. I encouraged, educated – almost begged – her to try taking an antidepressant medication, also an appropriate treatment for OCD. She declined. Steps towards recovery start by establishing trust – and this was difficult because of the degree of distraction and distress caused by Diedre's bombarding thoughts.

From Diedre, Macklin and Esmelda I learnt that deeply embedded, complex problems don't have easy or quick solutions. I learnt about the struggle that service providers have knowing what to do when well-intentioned efforts to encourage – or compel – adherence, for a person's own benefit, don't achieve the hoped-for results. I learnt about the risk of people, like Diedre, falling between the cracks in services. Or like Esmelda and Macklin, bouncing around in cross-referrals between different services – mental health, community geriatrics, drug and alcohol services – often coming up against a litany of reasons why a particular service is not the right place to provide care – arms held crossed in front of the service provider entry point announcing 'no deal', as if on some television game show.

❖❖❖

Sometimes, there were wonderful, heart-warming stories of hope.

It was impossible not to like Mimi and Joe. Both were in their late seventies, but Joe had a full head of hair, with only a smattering of grey. He maintained an active youthfulness that meant he seemed much younger than his years. Mimi, by contrast, was diminutive and delicate. Rheumatoid arthritis had insidiously distorted her joints, rendering her mostly confined to a wheelchair, walking only short distances at home. She relied heavily on Joe, and he obliged with adoring devotion. There was just the two of them, having been unable to have children.

I came to know Mimi and Joe when caring for Mimi in hospital, admitted with an acute and life-sapping depression that robbed her of the last of her limited movement. Catatonia – a form of depression in which the person's neurological responses to the world become severely restricted – wrapped like a constricting blanket around her. She could not eat or speak and appeared to be in a state of stupor much of the time. Joe, recognising that Mimi's condition was life-threatening, was distressed.

The treatment of choice in such situations is electroconvulsive therapy. ECT is the most misrepresented, misunderstood and maligned of medical treatments. For Mimi, it was life saving, and over several weeks she recovered, emerging from the immobilising fog of depression as a gentle woman with a warm sense of humour. Previously pallid, she regained a healthy colour, and added her own, with her favourite pink lipstick.

I witnessed Mimi and Joe's deep love, and loyalty to each other. It was not merely a relationship in which Joe did all the heavy lifting as Mimi's carer. Mimi's companionship and wit was as important as Joe's practicality and vigour. I visited them at home, welcomed in to see them functioning together like comfortable dance partners. From Mimi and Joe, I learnt that starry-eyed romance is not just the domain of the young; it can flourish in the face of chronic illness and disability. I was reminded also of the power of recovery.

❖ ❖ ❖

Then there was Jock, a man in his late seventies. How he had lived that long was a mystery. Over years he had drunk way more whiskey and smoked more cigars than was healthy. He'd made and lost a few fortunes betting on horses and dogs. He had the irascible charm of a larrikin and the charisma of an entrepreneur.

Jock had bipolar disorder. His life was a cycle of manic 'ups' – when he would drink more, gamble more, sleep (much) less and find himself in all sorts of compromising situations – and depressed 'downs', when he would disappear, racked with dark and deathly thoughts.

He was well acquainted with psychiatrists and had a long history of ambivalence regarding the medications intended to stabilise his mood, but which he found tended to cramp his style, like a chemical straightjacket. He felt much more alive when he was 'running high'.

When I knew him, he was red-faced, puffed and increasingly unable to live on his own. He had heart trouble, chronic breathing difficulties, problems with his memory, and he fell over frequently. He was in and out of hospital with medical problems, delirium and episodes of mania that were increasingly angry and irritable. In hospital he would throw food, insist on taking his pants off, and yell profane insults and demands at nurses, doctors and other patients. At these times, everyone struggled to view him with charity.

When not in hospital, Jock was still driving. He owned a once sleek but now worn sports convertible. One day he arrived at the community mental health centre wanting to see his favourite community nurse and drove right up to the door, stopping just centimetres before the glass. Bollards were put up within days to prevent such an event occurring again.

No doctor enjoys telling someone that they are no longer safe to drive – but it was necessary. Not only that, but Jock's deteriorating ability to make safe judgements resulted in an application to the Civil and Administrative Tribunal for appointment of a guardian from the Public Advocate. With escalating health problems and mishaps, his guardian decided he could no longer safely live by himself, and he was admitted to a residential aged care facility.

He was incensed at the loss of independence and unable to recognise his own limitations and the palpable dangers facing him, or others intersecting with him. As was his right, he appealed against the guardianship order and the special powers that placed him in care against his will. A lawyer was provided to represent him. His appeal was unsuccessful, given the mounting evidence of deteriorating function and capacity.

He remained in care, awkward and hostile towards most of the people around him, and took to writing prolific, vitriolic letters of complaint to any important person he could think of: members of the tribunal, the Chief Psychiatrist, the minister. In some of these letters I featured as 'Killer McKellar', the doctor who had wrongfully initiated his losses. Eventually, as Jock succumbed to worsening frailty, the letter writing ceased.

From Jock, I learnt about the tensions between respect for autonomy and duties of care. I learnt that the best efforts of health practitioners might not be understood by the person to whom they are directed, and may impact their sense of self and wellbeing – frequently with deep loss. In the shadow of these losses, I learnt not to take 'Killer McKellar' too seriously.

❖ ❖ ❖

Margie was, in some ways, like Jock. She was also in her mid-seventies and presented with contradictions between polarising moments of charm and challenge. I first met her on a community visit with another clinician. I knocked on the door of her tiny public housing unit in one of the disadvantaged far-northern Adelaide suburbs.

'Go away!' Margie yelled from within.

Eventually, she opened the door – heavyset, lumbering, angry, blustering and breathless. The more she talked, with unexpectedly articulate, socially superior intonation, expressing her outrage at our presence, the more cyanotically blue her face became, spreading from her lips to her nose across her cheeks, until she looked gravely unwell. Afraid she might have a cardiac event, I pleaded for her to come with us for a medical review, or to at least agree to visit her general practitioner. Being angry and refusing to see the doctor are not grounds for detention under the Mental Health Act, so when she slammed the door, we did not push her further.

Margie was born in Singapore to British parents, who later migrated to Australia. She grew up accustomed to privilege, attending elite schools and living in comfortable suburbs of Sydney, then Adelaide. She was a talented artist and as a young adult won a scholarship to study in Paris.

Somewhere along the line, things went wrong. She had relationships in which she was the victim of domestic violence. She drank heavily. At times she was the perpetrator of domestic violence. Her life became chaotic. She was unable to maintain her career, and after a series of questionable personal decisions, she sold the home she had inherited from her parents in one of Adelaide's most affluent suburbs.

When I met Margie, her money was gone and she was living in poverty, enraged at the world. I heard more of her story; the privilege of her early life tempered by the narrative of a punitive relationship with both parents. Her mother regularly beat and berated her for not living up to family expectations. It was not difficult to understand the genesis of Margie's skewed relationships.

Margie's life became a case study in the law of entropy. She was in and out of the hospital with multiple medical complaints and several suicide attempts. Wherever she went, the nursing staff had a terrible time – being yelled at with multiple demands and confronted by threats of self-discharge or further self-harm. Margie quickly became marginalised as a 'difficult patient', a particular type of 'other'.

I received stressed calls from the nursing staff on the medical ward. 'We need you to come and see *your* patient,' they demanded.

'She's *mental health*,' they would say, thereby indicating that her care was not really their business, and not seeming to realise how this categorisation was fundamentally dehumanising.

We'd never think to define another person, 'they're *cardiology*', as a point of identification, simply based on them having a heart problem. But Margie's interactions were so challenging that it was difficult for practitioners not to get caught in a cycle of rejection.

'She's a *full-on PD*,' people would say, referring to her diagnosis with a severe personality disorder, terminology that, when used pejoratively as it was here, offered little hope. The language of othering was embedded around Margie. Negotiating a therapeutic truce to navigate a way forward was extraordinarily challenging.

My working relationship with Margie ran hot and cold. At times I was her best friend – when she perceived I might serve some useful purpose to assist her. At other times, I was despised as another person to let her down or impose some harsh restriction on her.

Visits to the hospital were interspersed with trips to the Civil and Administrative Tribunal for debates over her capacity to make decisions for herself. For a while, Margie presented herself well and maintained the right to manage her affairs but struggled to sustain affairs at home.

After one hospital admission, having just won the right to be discharged from under the Mental Health Act and return home, she found herself so stressed by the challenges of independent life that she drove back to the hospital, took an overdose of paracetamol in the parking lot, and called the emergency department to tell them she was there.

Shortly after this, Margie's landlord evicted her from her accommodation. On a subsequent home visit, I found her living in a shared boarding house, in a room with a muscled and heavily tattooed man recently released from prison on one side, and a man dealing drugs on the other. The bathroom was shared and unable to accommodate the walking frame she required by then. It was the Adelaide summer and heading towards forty degrees. She had no air-conditioning and poor insulation. We found melting packs of cheese in Margie's room, reflecting her reluctance to use the shared kitchen.

She was readmitted to hospital. By this stage, the case for impairment in decision-making was clearer. Back in the tribunal, Margie was placed under guardianship (for her accommodation and care needs) and administration (of her limited financial affairs).

With no hope of Margie being accepted by a residential aged care provider, and unable to maintain independence in the community, a team decision was made to refer her for admission to Oakden, under the Mental Health Act, which was able to mandate that, for her, there was nowhere else to go.

Margie hated living at Oakden. She hurled abuse at the people she considered her captors – only reinforcing the view that she was rightly placed there. She broke windows. Like Jock, she wrote letters of complaint. She appealed, unsuccessfully, against her orders.

Eventually, matters settled down and she was accepted to move to a residential aged care facility. By the time the Oakden review took place in 2017, she was no longer there.

When I reflect on the decision-making process that led to Margie's admission to Oakden, I'm conflicted. She was caught in a system that was poorly able to meet her needs. Her behaviour was challenging, and frequently unacceptable. There were, literally, no quality options available for her.

I imagine what I might have encountered in a sliding-doors universe, that day I found her holed up in the boarding house. I might just as easily have found her dead in her room – either due to suicide or medical compromise. Did the possibility of this alternate ending make the journey down a pathway against her will more reasonable?

Margie's story had multiple threads: her early artistic talent and promise, her fear-inducing relationship with a harsh maternal figure, her later flawed decision-making and push-pull relationship with care providers. It was too easy to lose her human value in the theatre of her misadventure. The tragic lesson I learnt from Margie is that sometimes people's lives take turns from which they do not recover.

❖ ❖ ❖

Because of the intersection with my mother's story, I found natural connection with the people who came to see me in clinic concerned about memory changes. I would work through assessments with them, send them off for scans of their brains, and bring them back to clinic to jointly explore their unfolding stories.

Sometimes, I provided reassurance. Other times, I made a diagnosis. On some occasions, I was met with devastation, other times denial. One man, brought in by his family said to his daughter, 'Who's that person you took me to see? He's not a *real* doctor. There's nothing wrong with my memory. He just made that up. I'm not going back there again!'

Other times, having a diagnosis was a relief.

I saw Don and Mary, both in their late sixties. Mary had Crohn's disease, a chronic autoimmune disorder of the gastrointestinal tract. Throughout her years of illness, Don had been her primary support. Now Don presented with symptoms that looked like Parkinson's disease – tremor, falling over, shrinking handwriting. He also complained of a 'foggy brain', aware of his increasing difficulty remembering things and processing tasks he used to find easy. He was also struggling emotionally, feeling depressed, anxious and uncertain of the future. I brokered brain scans, neuropsychology reports and an opinion from a neurology colleague. At the same time, we worked together on Don's anxiety and mood.

There was agreement that Don was early in an illness that was causing progressive changes in his brain. It was likely that this was Lewy body disease, the third most common cause of dementia.

But Don and Mary were inherently positive people. They expressed gratitude for their lives, their three adult children and multiple grandchildren. They had made sensible – although modest – financial arrangements for retirement. They acted on plans to downsize their home and organise their life. They wrote advance care directives. They focused on healthy living, managing stress, and a good night's sleep. They thought about places they still wanted to see and refused to give up planning holidays.

Don and Mary taught me how people can live well with dementia, in control of their lives. They convinced me of the value of positive, hopeful conversations early in the illness, not simply making a diagnosis and letting people go off to sort things out by themselves.

❖ ❖ ❖

Elsewhere, when working on the acute mental health wards, I encountered people caught up in the trauma of difficult behavioural and psychological symptoms of dementia. Many, although not all, were men with younger onset dementia, often physically strong but with difficulty understanding their environments, communicating their needs, and managing emotions and behaviour. There is no doubt that neither acute medical nor traditional aged care environments are appropriate for the care of this group of people. Partly because of the inadequacy of care environments, styles of care, numbers and quality of staff, and partly because of the inherent nature of the symptoms themselves, situations occurred with real risk of harm.

While I was still in training, I met Boris, who was not yet sixty-five. He was tall, solid and strong. Because of dementia he was unable to control explosive bursts of agitation.

I vividly recall him holding a nurse up against a wall with his brawny forearm pressed against her neck. There was a terrifying hiatus in which time slowed down. Other staff moved to intercept the incident, trying not to make things worse. The situation was de-escalated without anyone experiencing physical harm, but the nurse was away from work, needing therapy following the trauma.

The situation was extraordinary – and thankfully vanishingly rare – but it would be an error to presume that such situations never occur. Dementia can be a highly complex illness.

Boris had treatment trials with various antipsychotics – medications that we know have limited value in the management of dementia, but sometimes can be helpful – providing they are reviewed, monitored and, when no longer needed, discontinued. Because of his age and the severity of his agitation and subsequent aggression, Boris received increasing doses.

Appearing to have no other option, he was referred to Oakden, where the doses of medication further increased. He experienced side effects, including becoming stiff and having difficulty walking, with his head awkwardly fixed in a forward nod. His illness progressed and his symptoms moderated. He died because of an infection, but it was never fully resolved how much the high-dose medications, or their side effects, contributed to his demise.

When Boris was sent to Oakden it was such a volatile situation that it appeared there was no alternative. Perhaps a different environment, and an approach that provided more time, space and personal interaction, may have eased Boris' symptoms more effectively. Sadly, hindsight is of no value to Boris.

Some years later, when I was working as a consultant at the Queen Elizabeth Hospital, I provided care for a retired businessman called Phil. He presented with advancing dementia, complicated by agitated and aggressive behaviour. His aged care facility had sent him to the hospital following repeated rampages, breaking windows and doors, and pushing other residents over. They were clear: they could not safely provide him care and would not have him back like this.

There was system pressure to discharge him. I started to think there was no alternative but to make a referral to Oakden, although by this time, I was aware that this would provide Phil unacceptable treatment.

One day, I was discussing Phil's care with a nurse on the ward, trying to work out how best to manage his constant drive to be up walking (therefore increasing his risk of falling).

'Well, at Oakden, that problem would be solved,' said the nurse, who had been a mental health nurse for many decades and had previously worked in long-stay wards like Oakden. 'They'd just sit him down and use a lap restraint,' he said.

I immediately recognised that, while this might manage a perceived difficulty for the service and secure a discharge, it would do absolutely nothing to relieve Phil's driving need to walk, would make him more agitated, and would rob him of quality of life.

I met with Phil's family and told them that, even though he could not, at that stage, return to his aged care facility, I was not prepared to make a referral to Oakden. We would just need to keep going, working out what Phil needed to feel more settled.

Phil remained in the hospital's care for numerous months, and the natural history of his illness followed its course. His walking deteriorated, as did his appetite and awareness of his surroundings. As frailty became more prominent, he was able to transition back to the facility, where he received tender, respectful care at the end-of-life.

After Phil died, I received a heartfelt message of thanks from his daughter, grateful that his life was honoured with dignity and kindness that pushed back against the pressure to 'flow' him out of the system he was in – a pathway that, had we followed it, would have led to his harm. It is true that we must manage the system to ensure we can meet the most needs in the best possible way – but we have to keep the person at the centre of care as we do this.

From Phil, I learnt that it is important to have the courage to do the right thing.

6

On the brink

Things seldom make sense in an instant. Sorting out what I was learning from the stories of older people, and people with challenges in their mental health or experiences of disability, occurred gradually. At the same time, I thought about how I could use this insight to make a difference in the world, aware that this vocational work would not occur single-handedly but through partnerships. Between 2014 and 2016, I became more concerned about what I had seen and heard of the service at Oakden and hoped that change would be inevitable. I just didn't know *how* this would occur. My convictions about Oakden became symbolic for me of broader issues in humanising health and social care.

When I started working in the older persons' mental health service, my new bosses asked me what I thought the strategic priority should be.

'Oakden,' I replied, thinking of my own observations and the perceptions I frequently heard from colleagues. 'We need to do something about Oakden.'

They did not disagree with this, but there were other priorities, and negligible resources. I now consider myself fortunate not to have been asked to work within Oakden at that time, as I would have found myself in a compromised position, with limited organisational support, confronted by an impoverished service culture, and not yet personally ready for the change process required. Oakden's problems were yet to come into the spotlight. Sometimes timing is critical.

Instead, I ended up working in a different region. This provided me with adequate independence to become part of the later Oakden review panel. I continued to watch and listen as services interacted around the goings on at Oakden. I found myself attending to stories told by a group of doctors, several of whom were yet to undertake postgraduate training, who were serially posted at Oakden during the last few years prior to the review.

These doctors felt overwhelmed. Sometimes they found themselves just hanging on until their limited terms of employment came to an end and they could get away. They were exposed to professional risk and reached out to others of us working elsewhere, debriefing, and seeking support. I received several calls.

'I don't think it's safe to work here,' one of the doctors said to me. 'I'm going to be held responsible for something that feels like it's beyond my control.'

'They call it time-out,' the same doctor later stated of the practice of shutting 'difficult' residents in empty parts of the facility, alone for hours and unattended to, 'but it's seclusion.' She felt inadequately equipped to escalate her concerns but knew there was a breach in legislation and human rights. 'I can't seem to get anyone to listen. I feel so alone.'

Another doctor recounted a story to me, shortly after she had escaped from her term at Oakden. She described how she had been preparing to finish for the day, just before five o'clock. One of the nursing staff spoke to her casually, as an aside.

'*So you're aware,*' they said, using a code for handing over responsibility to the doctor, 'we've just put Mr Digby in a side room. He's passing.'

'What do you mean he's passing?' the doctor asked.

'You know, he's passing. As in ... *passing away ...*'

'What? When did he become unwell? How come nobody let me know or asked me to review him?' The doctor was aghast.

The doctor rushed to review Mr Digby, who was unwell with a treatable infection. She contacted Mr Digby's family and commenced treatment. Mr Digby did not die. He recovered and was later discharged from Oakden to a more comfortable home. Not surprisingly, the doctor was very late home that day, and disturbed by the lack of capability in clinical assessment she had witnessed and the readiness to consider a life ready-for-disposal, without understanding what was going on.

Another one of the doctors recounted a story of how she had to dash to the supermarket to buy torches on a night when a severe storm caused a blackout over Adelaide. It was only in such a crisis that the absence of contingency planning became evident.

'I was worried that we would lose power,' the doctor told me. 'Lights were going out all over the city, but the staff still didn't want to help get the residents into bed. And then the lights went out and it was completely dark. It was terrible!'

The narratives from these medical staff, who tried their best to do the right thing but often ended up bunkering down just to survive, reinforced what I had learnt from my own observations and from the mutterings, complaints, and frustrated, fatalistic eye-rolling of colleagues and local aged care stakeholders: Oakden was a service with deep dysfunction. It was a ticking timebomb that no one with the power to change things seemed to be noticing.

During this period, armed with a sense of responsibility to advocate for action around the Oakden-shaped elephant in the room of South Australian mental health services, I took an opportunity to sit on the local branch committee of the Royal Australian and New Zealand College of Psychiatrists. The College is an independent professional body, responsible for setting standards for the training and qualification of psychiatrists as medical specialists. The South Australian branch committee provided a point of engagement with state government and the local community regarding mental health. It was a valuable schooling in policy, politics, and the need for persuasion to get things done. I took the role of representing the mental health needs of older people and the services providing care for them very seriously, and repeatedly raised the idea that the College should engage in lobbying for reform of the Oakden Campus.

On the brink

One thing leads to another, and because of my involvement with the branch committee, I took part in two delegations to South Australian state government ministers. On each occasion, my sole intention was to flag Oakden as a problematic service and to request that the ministers initiate a change-process by visiting the campus and becoming better informed about the people who lived there. My account of these meetings was later placed on the public record by Bruce Lander QC, in his report of the Independent Commissioner against Corruption, published in 2018.[1]

The first meeting was in 2014, with Jack Snelling, Minister for Health (and Mental Health), and his team. Leesa Vlahos, who later became Minister for Mental Health, was present at the meeting as the parliamentary secretary. There were several other representatives of the College of Psychiatrists in attendance, with a list of numerous issues. I was not the first to speak. Youth mental health, the trouble with emergency department wait times, these more pressing issues were higher up the agenda. When it was my turn, time was short, and I needed to get to the point. It was my first visit to a minister's office, and I tried to balance urgency with respect. Perhaps I did not speak plainly enough. But I did tell the minister that there were serious issues in the delivery of care to the highly vulnerable older people at Oakden and, unquestionably, someone from the minister's office needed to visit the site and take a concerted look at what was going on. The minister agreed. I innocently and sincerely believed that Mr Snelling and his team would act on this information.

When this encounter was later scrutinised by Bruce Lander, during his review, Mr Snelling stated that he 'did not have a memory of this meeting' and that he did not believe serious issues were raised about the quality of care being provided at Oakden.[2]

There is a lesson here: if you want to blow a whistle and get attention, you need the courage to be clear and loud enough to not be forgettable. Don't be so polite that no one gets the message. Older people are already invisible enough as it is. Despite my request and the minister's agreement that it was a good idea, there was no visit.

The second meeting was in late 2016, with Leesa Vlahos, who by that time had been promoted to Minister for Mental Health. Parliament was in session. The minister, along with many of her colleagues, had been up most of the night debating the euthanasia bill. She was clearly – and understandably – fatigued, and we were grateful that she had made the time to meet with our delegation from the College. I was concerned that I would not have time to make an adequate submission about Oakden, remembering the timidity and over-politeness of my first attempt. The Chair of the Branch Committee and Dr Aaron Groves, the Chief Psychiatrist, were both present in our group and, as usual, there was a list of issues to raise.

The minister graciously managed introductions and then sat to listen through our list. Once again, the people living at Oakden were not on top of the agenda. First came a petition to save the statewide gambling response unit, then concerns about child and adolescent mental health services. There were so many compelling needs jostling for patronage. When it was my turn, I tried to quickly convey the vulnerability of the people at Oakden, the under-resourcing of the service and the aberrant culture.

'Minister, there is illegal seclusion and restraint occurring at Oakden,' I blurted out.

This was entirely true. At that point, the minister raised her hand to stop me. I had an awkward moment of fearing that I had said the wrong thing.

The minister redirected the narrative, saying: 'I'll deal with that through the Chief Psychiatrist's office.'

I finished my submission by imploring the minister to organise a visit to Oakden to review the environment and the service.

'I will,' she said. 'Let me come and learn.'

I do not doubt that her intentions were sincere. Efforts were made to organise a visit, brokered by the College of Psychiatrists with the minister's office. I repeatedly checked in with the College secretariat to see what was happening but was frustrated by repeated delays and rescheduling.

On the brink

In the end, Minister Vlahos' visit did not materialise. Ironically, she remained unaware that the Oakden story was about to take over her life and change it irrevocably. Like a wave building strength before crashing against a rocky shoreline, events were taking on a momentum of their own. Barb Spriggs was persisting in seeking to tell her husband Bob's story and finally managed to gain an audience with the Northern Adelaide Local Health Network's CEO, Jackie Hanson. She also connected with Nicola Gage, a local journalist for the Australian Broadcasting Corporation. Circumstances teetered on the brink.

And then, a few days before Christmas in 2016, my phone rang. It was Aaron Groves.

'There's been a serious complaint about Oakden,' he said. 'A family member has met with Jackie Hanson and told their story.'

I was immediately engaged. Something was about to happen.

Aaron continued: 'Jackie's very concerned. She's already taking steps to make changes at Oakden, and she's commissioned me to undertake a review under the statutory powers of the Mental Health Act. I'm putting together a team to help me and I'd like you to be on it.'

'Absolutely,' I said without hesitation.

I earnestly believed that this was the most critical task in South Australian health and aged care history for many years and I was not going to miss the opportunity to make a difference.

'Of course,' I added, tempering my enthusiasm to remember due process, 'I'll request the appropriate clearances …'

I received approval and joined the Chief Psychiatrist's review of the Oakden Older Persons' Mental Health Service. I still consider it remarkable that I happened to be in that place at that time.

Collectively, those of us delivering health and social care were on the brink of an important uncovering about how we, as a system, were addressing the needs of older people experiencing complex vulnerabilities – people who too quickly became awkward *'others'* and sat outside of the mainstream concerns of health services. We were about to ask how our system and community leaders were managing accountability in relation to this – or, as it became clear, not managing.

AN EVERYONE STORY

On a personal level, the stories from my life and family, the tutelage of the 'teachers' I had provided care for as a doctor, and my growing exposure to how systems and services interact around human needs were coalescing. I was on the brink of expansive and ultimately life-transforming learning.

PART 2

Into the Breach

7

When the story is told

The Oakden Review commenced in January 2017, while most Australians were still enjoying the festive priorities of the summer slow-down. The review team gathered in the South Australian Department of Health for a briefing and explanation of the powers of investigation extended to us as delegates of the Chief Psychiatrist. These statutory powers, enshrined in the Mental Health Act, gave us permission to speak candidly about whatever we might find in the review, and in this way addressed a potential conflict of interest for those of us on the team who worked elsewhere for the Department of Health.

Aaron Groves, the South Australian Chief Psychiatrist, was the redoubtable leader of the process, frequently reminding us that when things got difficult due to our reporting of contentious issues, it was his review, and he would take responsibility for what we said. At the same time, he modelled democracy and collaboration, and we consistently felt like a team, with confidence that everyone was listening to each other.

The other team members were Del Thomson and Nicholas Procter. Del is a seasoned mental health nurse, grounded in wisdom, having witnessed the full spectrum of issues occurring in mental health services. Nicholas is Professor of Mental Health Nursing at the University of South Australia, able to balance warmth toward the individual with acumen for discerning the organisational and political landscape. Brett Coulson, a senior psychiatrist from Victoria, came across several times to assist with some of the politically sensitive interviews, adding another perspective. My place on the panel was as a local old age psychiatrist – and Aaron was aware of my earnest belief that something needed to be done about Oakden, having seen my attempt to initiate action from the Minister for Mental Health in our meeting just months before.

Aaron, as I came to know well, loves to talk and is not averse to a good drama. I have enough insight into my own proclivities to know that, in this way, we are kindred spirits. Histrionic potential aside, Aaron is a formidable workhorse. He has a keen mind, vast systems knowledge, and tremendous energy. He can maintain concentration and intensity for hours, driven to get to the bottom of issues and get things right. Numerous times, he saw Del and me flagging after our long sessions of discussion or reviewing documents and would send us home, while he remained at the office until late into the night: reading, writing, reflecting. In his leadership of the review, Aaron had honesty and integrity. I learnt a great deal from him, and he became a friend.

From the first moment, there was a sense of gravity to the work on which we were embarking. We all understood that this was an investigation that was years overdue. In the beginning, we were not even aware of a previous review undertaken by Simon Stafrace and Alan Lilly, two colleagues from interstate, a decade earlier.[1] Their report was buried somewhere in the Department of Health, with none of its recommendations having been implemented. Aaron uncovered this earlier work, and we were struck, first, by the synergy with our findings, despite the passage of time, and second, with a sense of outrage at opportunity lost. What does it take to get system-wide attention and secure real and lasting change?

What became apparent was that, in garnering system-wide attention, there is no more powerful medium than a gripping and powerfully told human story. The truth is, the Oakden review only occurred because Barb Spriggs was courageous and determined enough to tell her story – and did so with such efficacy that people listened.

When the story is told

By the time Barb Spriggs, supported by her children Clive and Kerry, met with the review panel to tell us her story first-hand, the burden of campaigning to expose what had happened to her husband, Bob, and what she was convinced was happening to others, had taken its toll. The strain of seven months of persistent agitation to be heard, and the public and political attention that was already mounting, had left her weary. Her meeting with the review panel was delayed while she travelled overseas with her family, seeking sanctuary and restoration, and still grieving the loss of her husband.

Important here is the fact that Bob Spriggs' story was not unique. It typified the trauma of many people and their families cornered into residence at Oakden. In telling Bob's story, Barb was measured and articulate. She described his diagnosis with younger-onset Lewy body dementia, complicated by Capgras syndrome – a psychiatric phenomenon where he had episodes of believing that Barb was another person, at which time he would become hostile and frightening towards her. She described how this became such a problem that she was not able to care for him at home, and so began his journey through hospital to Oakden. Her reasonableness and lack of drama, alongside her tenacity, were the very features that added weight to her narrative. As a result, her account became central to the case, and she became a spokesperson for many. For us as a panel, hers was one of numerous stories that surfaced during the review, stories that left us frequently shaking our heads and reeling with vicarious trauma.

❖ ❖ ❖

'It was a disaster from the word go,' Barb stated of Bob's admission to Oakden.

Bob had been in one of the acute older persons' mental health hospital wards before going to Oakden, with high levels of staff around him and the care of multiple health disciplines. He was well managed in that environment, and there was an awareness that he would not survive long in a mainstream aged care facility.

'We didn't want him to go to Oakden, but there appeared to be no choice,' Barb told us. 'Before he was sent there, we were told that Oakden was the only place in the state that he could go, and he couldn't stay in the hospital forever.'

Barb described her shock on arriving at Oakden. 'It looked derelict,' she said. 'We thought we were in the wrong place.'

The message from some of the senior staff, presumably to provide reassurance, was that Bob was privileged to have a place at Oakden. Barb was given a tour of the facility, including the activity area at the rear of the complex, only to later discover that Bob never gained access to that part of the site because he was considered too difficult to manage. Instead, he remained in Makk House, the men's area, devoid of personal comfort and meaningful interaction.

When Barb went to visit Bob on his second day, she found him dressed in someone else's clothes. Bob was an immaculate man, but at Oakden, Barb never saw him in his own clothes or dressed neatly. One day, Barb arrived and, when seeing a dishevelled figure in the distance, asked herself, 'Who's that person walking up and down over there?' As she got closer, to her horror, she discovered it was Bob. Another time, she found Bob lying on his bed, naked except for a continence aid. 'It looked like he was in a nappy,' she said. Even the bed – which was the only furniture in the austere room – was stripped back to just one sheet. After Bob had left Oakden, Kerry returned to pick up his clothes. She was handed a garbage bag full of items; none of them belonged to Bob.

Barb visited Oakden every day during Bob's time there. She began deliberately visiting at different times, so the staff would not know when to expect her. She had lost trust almost immediately and hoped, by arriving unannounced, to find out what was really going on. Often, she would arrive at the ward to find no staff visible. On one occasion, another visitor, already on site, told her Bob had fallen and been left slumped over a chair for a long time before anyone had come to help. Another time, Barb found Bob lying on the floor, alone in his room with the door closed. She had no idea how long he had been there.

The family were told that Bob had difficulty accepting food and fluids. One day, Bob's son Clive found him distressed and repeating the same dry-lipped syllable over and over: 'Phew ... phew ...' Clive realised that Bob was thirsty and was trying to communicate that he needed a drink. He had no difficulty helping his dad take a drink. It seemed to Clive that the staff were not checking in to make sure Bob was offered a drink. Another day, it took Clive twenty minutes to find a staff member when he recognised that Bob was thirsty and uncomfortable and needed help with changing his continence aid.

Another time, Barb turned up to visit Bob and saw a nurse feeding him, only to discover them 'shovelling in the chocolate pudding' without dignity or care. By the time he left Oakden for the last time, Bob was severely dehydrated and malnourished.

Bob could become highly agitated and aggressive. Staff were afraid of him. Barb was informed that Bob had 'exposed himself' to one of the nurses, suggesting that he had done this intentionally to be inappropriate and was somehow 'bad'. Intuitively, she understood that the staff saw Bob as the problem, as if his behaviours were a deliberate act rather than a consequence of his illness. His experience exemplified the *othering* of the person with dementia.

The situation deteriorated and Bob was secluded in a locked area at the end of the men's unit, which in summer became excessively hot. 'He would have been better off in jail,' Barb told the review panel.

When Bob had arrived at Oakden, he was able to talk. Barb had concerns over the medications used to manage his symptoms and felt frustrated trying to get information about this. She learnt that an error had occurred in which he had been repeatedly administered ten times the dose of antipsychotic he should have been prescribed. 'All I know,' she stated, 'was that after two days at Oakden he had lost his ability to speak.' She was worried that medications contributed to this.

One day, when Barb arrived to visit Bob, she found him sitting on the floor, with two nurses standing over him. She was unsure what was going on. 'We're just about to change him,' one of the nurses told her. Barb noticed tears rolling down Bob's cheeks. He looked at her imploringly, unable to communicate in words. 'I believe he was afraid,'

Barb stated. 'There was something about what was happening that made him feel unsafe.'

Barb told us that she was never asked to provide consent for the use of restraints at Oakden. Nonetheless, Bob was confined to a chair with a lap restraint on numerous occasions.

Sometimes restraints were more subtle. During one visit Barb noticed Bob struggling to stand up from a deep wingback chair. She could sense his frustration.

'He's having trouble getting out of the chair,' she told a staff member.

'Exactly,' she was told, 'that's why we put him there.'

Kerry was visiting one day and felt uncomfortable when her dad kept trying to pull his pants down to expose his upper leg. She encouraged him to settle but then was shocked when she noticed the deeply coloured and expansive bruise across his pelvis and leg. It dawned on her that he was trying to communicate with her. He had been injured and was in pain.

It was the final straw for the family. They believed the bruise had been caused by a restraint, against which Bob had struggled. No formal record of the restraint was found. The review panel learnt that a lone chair with a lap restraint attached to it had been found in the area where Bob was kept in seclusion. The photograph of this bruise, taken by Bob's family, became one of the often-published media images, illustrating the standard of treatment at Oakden.[2]

'The photo didn't do it justice,' Barb told the review panel. 'And when we met with the doctors, they were not even aware of it.'

The senior clinical team at Oakden realised that they were unable to provide adequate care for Bob. He was sent back to the acute ward from where he had come, with the assertion that he needed reassessment and further acute management. A short while later, with the enduring pressure to maintain service flow and empty beds in the hospital, the family was told that Bob would be sent to Oakden for a second time.

Separately, the review heard that an appeal against sending him back to Oakden was made by Oakden's medical officer, citing the inability of the service to provide safe care. The medical officer told the review panel that she did not receive a response to her emails from anyone in management.

Bob was sent back, and the horrible cycle occurred again, ending with Bob's seclusion, restraint, dehydration and deterioration. He was sent by ambulance to the Royal Adelaide Hospital, severely unwell. Remarkably, with antibiotics and fluid resuscitation he picked up, only for the doctor looking after him to say, 'By Monday he'll be ready to go back to Oakden – he can't stay here and there's no alternative.'

Barb was distressed. How could anyone think that Bob should go back to Oakden a third time? A nurse had overheard the interaction with the doctor and approached Barb and the family. Arrangements were made for Bob to be transferred back to the hospital ward he had come from in the beginning. When he got there, his speech improved, and he appeared calm and settled. Barb described Bob's interaction with one his favourite nurses on the ward. When he saw her for the first time after returning, his eyes welled with tears and, with hands outstretched, he smiled and whispered, 'My friend ...'

A tipping point had been reached. After a few weeks back on the ward it was evident that Bob would not fully recover. He was transferred to a hospice, where he died a short while later. Dementia is, ultimately, a terminal illness. Still, it is clear that Bob Spriggs' journey towards the end-of-life was fraught with unnecessary hardship due to a system that was not fit for purpose.

For Barb, Clive and Kerry, the arduous battle to tell his story and advocate for change was just beginning.

❖ ❖ ❖

There were other stories. As a review panel, we shared a sense of the cumulative burden of these narratives. Some of the families, encouraged by Barb Spriggs' courageous whistleblowing, also spoke publicly.[3]

Jim Baff was admitted to Oakden in 2014. His wife, Lorraine, described him as a 'gentle giant'. The former bricklayer was tall and strong and, an ex-rugby league player, he had taken some beatings on the football field. Jim also carried the impact of loss and trauma early in his life. Following the tragic death of his father when Jim was eight, his mother, devastated and unable to recover, left him to be raised by his older sister, Sandra, and his grandparents. He loved his sister and grandmother but struggled to overcome his mother's abandonment.

He'd wanted to go to university to become an accountant but was compelled to take an apprenticeship to make ends meet. Jim built a career in construction and, together with Lorraine, raised a devoted family, with children Warren and Trisch. He studied education as a mature-age student and established a successful business training people for the building industry.

Lorraine noticed changes in Jim's personality and abilities in his early fifties. In six months, he lost the ability to send an email. At fifty-six, he was diagnosed with Alzheimer's disease and life changed completely.

Trisch moved back to Adelaide to help look after her dad, living in a unit that Jim had built at the back of the family home. It had been his last project, completed with his son's help. It was here that Jim sought solace from his growing confusion, sitting with Trisch and telling her snippets of stories from his life, or poring over his extensive coin collection.

Jim became more troubled. He would frequently mistake Trisch for his sister, Sandra. At other times he would pack a bag and ask for help to go and find his mother. He had difficulty communicating and, increasingly frustrated, became irritable and demanding. He couldn't understand why he could no longer drive. He wandered away from home and was found kilometres away, alone and afraid. He locked the carers who came to help outside the house. When things didn't go how he wanted them to, he flared in anger.

'He would just go into these blind rages,' Lorraine explained. 'He literally ripped the security screen off the back door and tied it into a bow.'

When the story is told

Just as Barb Spriggs had done, Lorraine and Trisch cared for Jim at home for as long as they could. Lorraine became so stressed that her health deteriorated. Eventually it became evident that it was no longer safe for him or them.

He was admitted to a residential aged care facility in 2013 and, not surprisingly, it did not go well. Lorraine and Trisch would hear him pounding on the locked facility door as they left their visits. He became violent and destructive, and so was sent to hospital, where a cycle began with restraint, sedation and, when things improved, discharge back to the facility – only to be sent to hospital again when things deteriorated. Eventually, after a period of assessment and trials of various medications, he was placed under a guardianship order and referred to Oakden. There were no other options.

Lorraine was concerned from Jim's first moments at Oakden. She was taken aback by the environment, which she compared to a nineteenth-century asylum. 'It was so old and dilapidated, and the ceiling had stains all over it from possums,' she reported.

She tried to draw attention to the problems at Oakden. In 2014, she wrote to the state Minister for Health, whose office later stated they had no record of her letter. She visited her local member of parliament, agitating for action. 'Someone's going to get killed in that place,' she said.

The MP wrote to the minister, communicating Lorraine's concerns about the number and quality of staff. Parliamentary Secretary, Leesa Vlahos, wrote back, pointing out that the staffing levels at Oakden were higher than in other aged care facilities, and that the staff were specialists in managing challenging needs. From Lorraine's perspective, this provided no reassurance. She was witnessing the realities of life at Oakden.

Jim's condition declined. He experienced side effects to his medications. With no engagement in interesting activities, he deteriorated, losing his ability to walk unaided. He spent his days sitting in the same chair, in the same position, looking away from the window so that he could not see the outside world, bare as the landscape around Oakden was. He was almost continuously restrained. Having lost most of his language skills, he would call out in distress with a booming voice.

Then, in 2015, Lorraine received a phone call from one of the managers at Oakden, telling her that Jim had been assaulted by a staff member. 'We suspect it's not the first time,' Lorraine reported the manager telling her.

It had taken considerable courage for the junior staff to come forward and speak up against a senior, long-standing registered nurse. They reported witnessing the nurse stomp on Jim's legs, whilst he was restrained in a wheelchair.

Lorraine was furious. With Trisch, she rushed to Oakden, only to be reassured that the matter would be dealt with internally. Then, another nurse quietly slipped Trisch a piece of paper with the name of the nurse involved. Lorraine and Trisch went to the police station and reported the incident themselves. It took two years to get to court. The nurse pleaded guilty to aggravated assault and received a good behaviour bond, with no conviction.[4] No one spoke to the family again about what had happened, and they only learnt of the outcome incidentally. Trisch rang the minister's office twice to see if there would be any follow up and, on one occasion, the minister's staffer said, 'This case is going to be a big deal.' She never heard back from them.

Trisch was heartbroken by Jim's experience. Lorraine, unable to reconcile her guilt for having exposed him to Oakden, was stymied to have had no choice.

❖❖❖

There were other stories of rough-handling and assault.

One day, in December 2013, when Rina Serpo was visiting her eighty-two-year-old husband, Ermanno, as she did every day that he was at Oakden, she witnessed a staff member assault him. It appeared to her that Ermanno felt intimidated by the carer but, unable to communicate because of the disability caused by dementia, he raised his fists defensively at the carer. Rina reported that the carer grabbed Ermanno by his T-shirt, at his throat, and compelled him along the corridor, appearing to 'throw' him down onto a couch.

Like Lorraine Baff, Rina and her family were outraged – but not only because of the assault.

'There were instances when I couldn't find him,' Ermanno's daughter reported. 'He'd be in the courtyard in the middle of winter in a T-shirt and no shoes.' On numerous occasions she found faeces in the courtyard, or urine in the hallway, only to find that staff were aware but had not cleaned it up.

Ermanno's family also believed that medication was used to manage his behaviours by default, reflecting the limitations in the environment, the lack of other strategies and resources, and the general cultural mindset of staff. The family found him sedated, unable to eat or walk safely. They felt frustrated when they tried to escalate concerns about his clinical deterioration, feeling dismissed, and being told 'he's just tired'. Ermanno's daughter stated that sometimes, 'he'd walk to a corner and just look at a wall'.[5]

❖ ❖ ❖

Dawn, the steadfast mother of Kathy, who was living at Oakden with younger onset frontotemporal dementia due the C9orf72 gene, told how she would come to visit and find Kathy locked up, in a back section of the campus, roaming around the space alone. 'She was in a corridor area, with the light on at one end, with a chair and a table, that's all,' she said, frustrated by the deprivation. 'And she was always dressed terribly.'

One day Dawn arrived to collect Kathy to take her on an outing. Kathy hadn't eaten lunch, so Dawn thought it reasonable to wait. She got locked in with Kathy. They waited, but lunch never came. She knocked on the door and called out to the staff, with no response. Eventually, Dawn rang the front desk to get someone to come and let them out. 'Lunch finished an hour ago,' she was told, as if it were her error.

'I was always writing letters about things like that,' Dawn stated, 'but nothing changed.'

❖❖❖

These accounts from families were not outliers. Their experiences were echoed repeatedly throughout the review.

The review panel invited a group of about thirty family members of residents of Oakden to a meeting at the Office of the Public Advocate, deemed neutral ground. The Public Advocate and Chief Nurse attended, in addition to the review panel members. The utilitarian public meeting room was full, overhung by palpable anger and grief, juxtaposed with the tentative expectation and hope of change. CEO Jackie Hanson opened the meeting and then left, so as not to compromise families' freedom to speak plainly. Before this meeting, I had not met Jackie Hanson. She looked weighed down and had been away from work with shingles – an illness to which people succumb at times of extreme stress. Aaron Groves facilitated the discussion, which quickly took on a heart-wrenching life of its own as family members allowed their stories to tumble out.

Family members told the review they believed Oakden was the 'end of the road' – a place for people whose problems were so onerous that there was nowhere else for them. Families were already desperate, having been on the merry-go-round of multiple unsuccessful attempts at placement in aged care. Many had borne the brunt of their family member's aggressive behavioural symptoms themselves. They carried love, fear, responsibility and despair, while also carrying the bruises, scratches and pinch marks of having tried to deliver care at home.

Families felt powerless to question what they were told by the range of service providers they encountered on their odyssey through aged care, acute services and into Oakden. With no other choice available, they found themselves uncomfortably ambivalent, relieved to have paused the circumvolving search for care, but troubled by the evident deficits.

One family summed this up:

When the story is told

*The hospital told us there was nowhere else to go except Oakden;
when we got there the Oakden staff said there was nowhere else for
him to go except Oakden; but how can there be nowhere else to go?*

The demoralising message spoke to the value our community placed
on older people with complex needs. So prominent was this as a theme
within the stories, that we considered subtitling the report, 'Nowhere
else to go.'

The families also described an environment that was dark,
discomforting and depreciated – a neglected wasteland. One family
member told the review that 'Oakden is one of the most depressing
places you can visit'.

Our scouring of the campus supported their descriptions. Large
stains on the ceiling tiles provided evidence of Lorraine Baff's claims
about possums marauding in the roof. Gardens were left untended,
with dried weeds clogging disused beds. Deep cracks formed crazed
patterns across the parched earth. There was cheap, broken furniture.
There were curtains hanging by only half of their attachments and
leaking pipes encrusted with exudate. Paint was applied so long ago
that the walls had yellowed as if jaundiced. There were rumours of
infestations of foxes and fleas in catacombs beneath the building.
Families knew that their relatives were living in substandard
accommodation where there was an inadequate application of budget
for essential maintenance, let alone improvement.

Doors to gardens were frequently locked, the rationale being
that the uneven pavers were a falls hazard. Residents were confined
indoors, and the exterior grounds ran to rack and ruin. Families
and visitors arrived at a second-rank entrance – converted as a cost-
saving front door after the decommissioning of the original front of
the building – compelled to wander past the noisy plant room and, at
times, the pumping of the septic tank.

Incredulous, one family member told the review: 'And then there's
the septic! It's still on septic. They don't want to spend the money.'

A mantra of impoverishment set the tone for everyone at Oakden.

One family member recounted a conversation with one of the managers, saying:

> The manager was sympathetic to the issues we raised about getting more staff, better resources, but said, 'No money, no money.' They did not push the need for more staff any further. It was not considered a priority to push.

Futility settled over the service, stealing hope of change. Even the standard of catering reflected this. In the early days, cooking occurred onsite, offering the possibility of the warming smells of cooking and baking. It ceased as a cost rationalisation long before the review, by which time there was no cooking onsite – not even as a recreational or therapeutic activity. Meals were outsourced, delivered cold to the site from a commercial kitchen. Families complained that food was warmed up only to go cold again by the time it was served to the residents. 'It's stone cold,' a family member stated.

A scarcity of human engagement echoed the environmental poverty. Families complained that they would come in, particularly after hours, and be unable to find a staff member. Staff may have been busy attending to a resident in a bathroom, but the other residents were left unobserved, and families felt troubled and isolated by this.

One family member said that their relative had 'sat in wet pads while eating because no staff were available to change him'.

'There was no one around,' said another. 'We had to help residents and stop people ending up in an altercation.'

Deprivation included the marked lack of stimulation and engagement for residents. The activities area was a large room at the back of the campus, which in early years had offered a thriving hub of activity for the first residents. Years later, by the time of the review, the program had deteriorated. The remaining team of demotivated 'diversional therapy' staff predominantly confined their activity to that one room, requiring residents to come to them. Activities were typically not taken out to the ward areas where residents spent their time. Most residents were either unable, or unsupported, to leave the wards, where they remained, 'wandering', or reclined in princess chairs, deprived of engagement.

During a day of review at Oakden, I encountered one resident sitting by himself at a table in a room adjacent to the activities area. It was another cavernous, sparsely furnished space with undecorated red-brick walls. The diversional therapist, with limited communication skills, who appeared uninterested and poorly equipped for her job, had given the man two small unpainted wooden animals to play with – old homemade children's toys. He sat alone at a large table, facing the wall, perseverating as he repeatedly rubbed the ridge of the small wooden rabbit he had been given, starved of comfort or connection.

The stories conveyed by families, supported by our observations as a review panel, left no doubt: Oakden was depleted, beaten down, stripped bare and devoid of hope. It had lost its way. People and their families were left discombobulated and disempowered.

This was summarised by a family member who told the review, 'I leave the ward and feel scared for my husband.'

The families' stories also exposed a culture of dehumanisation and loss of dignity. At one end of the spectrum, this was reflected in stories of finding their relative looking unkempt, dressed in other people's clothes. Some families told the review that they had discovered their relative wearing clothes belonging to someone of the opposite gender. Other families said they had looked at the labels on clothing only to find that their family member was wearing the clothes of someone who had died. No defence regarding the busyness of staff or the complexity of the residents could alleviate the indignity of these experiences. Untidy, mismatched, dirty, covered in food and wearing someone else's clothes – these were typical descriptors of residents at Oakden.

One family member told the review:

They put him in someone else's clothes. He was staggering around the corridor in revolting clothes. A man with mental problems – stripped of his own clothes, without his own clothes. 'Where are his clothes?' I would ask. 'They are getting labelled,' was the reply.

This went on for weeks. The day he left Oakden, he left still wearing someone else's clothes. He was a proud man. He was proud of his appearance.

Similarly, family members stated that belongings went missing. One family had brought in perfume; within days it was nowhere to be found. Others brought in cash, stored in a cashbox with a ledger. Disappearances from the cashbox were unaccounted for and, even after being raised by the review panel, remained a mystery.

The families felt betrayed and trapped. The mismanagement of residents' personal belongings may not have amounted to direct physical harm but was indicative of dehumanised treatment. The point might be raised that there are illustrations of this in many aged care settings – as became evident in the stories told to Australia's Royal Commission. This only serves to underpin the importance of the Oakden story. The fact that older people might be treated as less than human *anywhere* should be a rallying call for compassionate, humanised care *everywhere*.

At the extreme end of the spectrum, just as the Spriggs, Baffs and Serpos had described, families told of neglect, malpractice, rough handling and abuse. One family member stated:

I have visited after hours on many occasions, and I have seen some disgusting things – things that should never happen.

Others helped explain these sentiments. A family member described finding faecal matter in their mother's hair, when coming to take her out. Another described their discovery of their family member receiving assistance with hygiene:

My father was in the toilet, and there were two male nurses, one on either side of him, each with a foot on his foot and holding his wrists. A female nurse started to clean him from behind, and he was startled and tried to get up – he was embarrassed.

When the story is told

❖❖❖

Oakden didn't only provide accommodation for people with dementia. One of the residents was a woman in her seventies called Vera, who was living with a diagnosis of schizoaffective disorder, an illness with features of both psychosis and depression. Vera was Dutch and, although she had been in Australia since the 1960s, her accent retained strong overtones from her childhood home. Vera had a sharp mind and, when she was well, could play (and win) a multiplicity of card games while holding a stiff poker face.

Vera had experienced severe trauma during her childhood that was tragically repeated after her arrival in Australia, including multiple sexual assaults. During the 1970s, she became pregnant after an assault and, in the devastating wake of her trauma and a subsequent miscarriage that compounded her losses, she became depressed, then psychotic, and never fully recovered. Her life became increasingly chaotic, and she spent more time in a hospital than living in the community. By the time she arrived at the Oakden Campus, she had been living in state mental health extended care services for two decades.

Vera found solace in her enduring love of animals. At Oakden, she could not have a pet, so she collected several fluffy toy dogs that she lined up in her room, speaking to them as if they were alive. At times, when she became acutely psychotic, the themes of lost autonomy and personal invasion were prominent and she would strenuously defend any attempt made by the staff to move her animals, even just to clean around them.

'Don't touch them!' she would scream, 'They're mine!'

It's not difficult to draw the connection between Vera's history of trauma and her aversion to any intervention, including assistance with personal hygiene. During the review, we learnt of Vera's experience of being compelled to take a bath. She would often decline to accept staff helping her with daily routines, despite struggling to manage her own continence. The review heard of times when staff would don face masks and protective clothing, to avoid Vera's spitting, and frogmarch her to the bathroom, insistent that it was time for her to take a bath.

She would spit and scream but could not prevent herself from being undressed and placed in the tub. Four staff would hold Vera while a fifth would quickly wash her.

We understood that, when Vera was unwell, it was difficult to work with her, but we could also see that her defensiveness was a product of years of institutional living in which she had been disempowered and retraumatised. Viewed and treated as the problem – the unquestionable 'other' – she was less than a person. Her experience might have been lifted from the pages of a Dickensian novel.

❖ ❖ ❖

Just as Lorraine and Trisch Baff had done, another family learnt that their relative had been assaulted during a meal. Like the Baffs, they were assured that matters would be managed 'in-house'. They came up against barriers when trying to report the incident to police and get a response to their concerns. Evidence is a vital requirement to progress an allegation. Despite another staff member and the man, himself, consistently maintaining the allegation, the outcome of the investigation was that there was insufficient evidence to confirm what had happened. The resident was living with a dual diagnosis of dementia and a mental illness. He was under guardianship and had been determined as having an impairment in decisional capacity. This did not mean that he could not express preferences, or, for that matter, accurately recall and describe events, but the nature of his disability meant that police advised there was no viable way for the case to progress. Understandably, the man's family felt an acute sense of injustice, as did the man himself.

It was the nature of the dysfunction at Oakden prior to publication of the report – secrecy from within, a lack of interest from without, and a lack of expertise within the organisation regarding how families might be supported – that no one was advised of their right to pursue civil damages claims when there were no criminal prosecutions in relation to assaults. In the months after the report's publication, in the reaction to previous inactivity, numerous staff were stepped down, multiple police reports made, and reports made to the health practitioners' regulation agency. Ultimately, a number of families were paid compensation.

In the first few months after the release of the Oakden Report, the health network was inundated with hundreds of complaints. People who had thought they were long since finished with their family experiences of Oakden came forward, their wounds freshly reopened by public reporting, wanting to tell their stories, having realised they were not alone in what they had been through.

❖❖❖

In the most disturbing story told during the meeting at the Office of the Public Advocate, a family member recounted an incident where a woman had been administered an 'in-out' catheter, to obtain a urine specimen. Consent had not been gained for the procedure. The woman had a known history of suffering domestic violence and assault. In an horrific turn of events, the wrong type of catheter was used – a wide-bore catheter intended for a male – and the procedure was aborted only after causing trauma to the woman, who was left distressed and bleeding. The event became the subject of a detailed investigation, the aftermath of which continued for several years. By the end of the family member's account of the incident, everyone in attendance was shell shocked. I looked across the room and saw the Chief Nurse weeping.

❖❖❖

We were told the story of a man called Ben, with complex needs, who had a psychotic illness that responded poorly to medical treatments. He was also slowly dying due to a chronic, progressive medical condition. He shuffled along with a four-wheeled walker, stooped over, with the frame running away in front of him until he fell over. He often became highly anxious, and people found his behaviour bizarre. He would lie on the floor and avoid speaking. Rather than engaging with him to check he was all right, staff would dismiss him as having 'floor time' and step around him. Ben was marginalised in health services because he looked eccentric and behaved in ways that people found unusual.

It is vital to acknowledge that there were caring staff within the system at Oakden, struggling to make a difference in the neglected backwater. Ben found a champion in the medical officer. Given that there were no occupational therapy staff, the medical officer took it upon herself to start a gardening club in one of the few unlocked, but still abandoned, garden areas. With no resources, besides a few cuttings and self-purchased seeds, she went outside with Ben, and they planted vegetables.

Over the months, like a secret garden awakening, seedlings flourished and turned into productive plants. When he went outside, Ben was transformed. The doctor discovered that Ben knew the names of the local bird species, recognising them not just by sight but also by their call. Instead of shuffling and falling, he would put his frame aside and walk securely between the vegetable beds, pushing his hands into the earth, turning his face toward the sunshine. In this unlikely and momentary deviation from the Oakden status quo, there was a glimpse of how the facility might have operated if its residents were released to the open air, with their humanity returned. But it was not to be sustained.

One day, the doctor and Ben went to the garden intending to harvest the zucchinis that were burgeoning in the raised beds. They were both dismayed to find their precious produce gone, neatly cut off at the stems. The mystery was never solved.

Ben was heartbroken. He wrote a letter to an unknown person in power far away from the world in which he lived, pleading to be released from Oakden. At the end of the letter, he captured the sentiment of all residents of Oakden: a simple drawn image of a bird escaping its cage.

8

Stories of place and time

People have stories. Places have stories too. Understanding the human stories that unfolded at the Oakden Older Persons' Mental Health Service requires context. Moreover, before we give attention to the stories of Oakden staff, and consider lessons regarding the deterioration of organisational culture, there are issues of place and time that warrant exploring.

Oakden didn't just happen. The scandal that erupted in 2017 was decades – even longer – in the making. It occurred because of multiple intersecting factors, including the place and time in which the events transpired, emerging from historically grounded institutional and clinical traditions. This context reflects the evolving perceptions of mental illness and dementia in Western communities over time, through generations. It reflects how services have developed and devolved while addressing the needs of people who encounter life-affecting conditions resulting in complexity and vulnerability. When it comes to the plight of people living with dementia or challenges in their mental health, the history of misunderstanding and marginalisation is deeply embedded.

Difficulties in mental health have been part of human experience throughout history. Ancient cultures proffered different explanations for mental illness, ranging from belief in possession by evil spirits to more physiologically informed views regarding the imbalance of life forces and bodily humours.[1] Dementia has had an intertwining relationship with mental disorders over time. The origin of the term is in the Latin *demens*, meaning 'to be out of one's mind'. There have been all sorts of words and descriptions for people living with dementia. Terms such as 'foolishness', 'idiocy', 'dotage', 'imbecility of the elderly', 'drivelling' and 'senility' have coloured the way dementia has been regarded, and placed people with dementia as outsiders, beyond the pale. The term *dementia* was used more commonly after the nineteenth century, after Philippe Pinel, the famous French alienist, used it specifically concerning cognitive changes of older age.[2]

In 2013, the *Diagnostic and Statistical Manual of Mental Disorders: Fifth Edition*, put forward a new terminology: major neurocognitive disorder. Underpinning this was recognition of the stigmatisation – the *othering* – experienced by people living with dementia through the ages, and an effort to move toward more clinically accurate language. For now, the term dementia remains embedded in our language. Perhaps the emphasis needs to be on ensuring that it is not used negatively. By giving people living with dementia respect, choice, empowerment and compassionate care, we can provide dignity to the terminology.

❖ ❖ ❖

The treatment of people with dementia, and people with mental illnesses, in care and place over time, makes for a sobering tale. Treatments have included all sorts of interventions, from exorcisms and religious rituals to trephination – the making of a borehole in the skull – and use of herbal medications and hallucinogens, bloodletting, fasting and starvation, cold baths and exercise – some of which were helpful; others, clearly, that were not.

In the earliest contexts, people with dementia or mental disorders were cared for by their families. Islamic hospitals cared for people with mental illness during the eighth and ninth centuries, with some degree of humanity and kindness in many cases. But, for the most part, the history of institutional care has been one of dehumanisation. Throughout much of Western history people with dementia and mental illness populated prisons. By the Middle Ages, 'madhouses' accommodated a conglomeration of people, most stricken by poverty. Patients might find themselves chained, beaten, or even presented as a source of public entertainment. In London in the sixteenth century, the public could pay to view the 'mad' incarcerated in Bethlem Hospital. Overcrowding, under-resourcing and poor treatment are themes that emerge again and again.

There are critical points in history where reformers surfaced. Pinel was successful in transforming prison environments to asylums – which in their name, at least, aspired to be places of refuge and sanctuary. The chequered history of the asylum movement reflects the struggle between aspirational, reformational goals and the social, political and economic realities of sustaining an institutional model. There were advocates and reformers such as Dorothea Dix. She campaigned for humane and benevolent treatment of people with mental illness – the 'indignant insane' – through the establishment of the first generation of public asylums in the United States during the mid-nineteenth century.

Contemporaneous with Dix was psychiatrist, administrator and architectural advocate Thomas Story Kirkbride, who led the well-intentioned expansion of the American asylum movement through the building of technologically advanced, expansive buildings to provide ongoing accommodation to the population with mental illness. Central to his belief was the idea that natural light, circulating air and access to beautiful landscapes and farming land was integral to the healing of mental illness.[3]

By the end of the nineteenth century, inadequate evidence of recovery for people living in institutional environments prompted doubts regarding the efficacy of the model. Psychiatry and psychoanalytic practices started moving away from institutional settings. By the time the Second World War was over, the asylum model was considered inhumane and ineffective and the gradual transition toward predominantly community-based models began.

AN EVERYONE STORY

❖ ❖ ❖

The story of people with mental illness in South Australia is grounded in this broader history. When British free settlers established the province as a colony in 1836 there was no other provision, so 'lunatics' were accommodated in a ward set aside within the Adelaide jail. In 1845, the Colonial Surgeon, Dr James Nash, raised concerns about this population with the Colonial Governor, only to be told that there were no funds available for more suitable accommodation. In response to mounting public pressure, a small number of inmates were relocated to a house in a local community called Parkside. Still, most remained in the prison until the Adelaide Lunatic Asylum was opened on North Terrace, one of Adelaide's main streets, in 1852.[4]

There was some subsequent expansion of the asylum, but overcrowding and substandard conditions continued to be a problem. In 1864, South Australia had its first formal review into a mental health service, which recommended the development of a new, purpose-built facility at the site of the Parkside cottage, away from the central city. The Parkside Lunatic Asylum was opened in 1870. Patients continued to be transferred from the Adelaide Lunatic Asylum until it closed, in a cloud of shame due to its squalid conditions, in 1902.

In 1913, the South Australian parliament passed the Mental Defectives Act, which defined people with a mental illness and those with an intellectual disability as 'defective'. At the same time, in a step toward increased enlightenment, the Parkside Lunatic Asylum changed its name to the Parkside Mental Hospital. Disturbingly, in 1931, the *Medical Journal of Australia* published an article arguing for the sterilisation of all people deemed 'mentally defective'.

The 1960s showed glinting promises of change in services for people with mental health conditions in South Australia, assisted by the arrival of Dr Bill Cramond OBE from Aberdeen in Scotland, a distinctive reformer and advocate for humane care who was unafraid to challenge the status quo. In 1964, the *Mental Health Amendment Act* finally differentiated between mental illness and intellectual disability.

In 1967, the Parkside Mental Hospital took a further step forward and changed its name to Glenside Hospital, operational to the present day in contemporary buildings, now called Glenside Health Services.[5] The impressive heritage buildings at the heart of the Glenside Campus, with touches of Kirkbride grandeur, were repurposed in 2011, as the South Australian Film Corporation studios, and the site of a leading art school. At its peak in the 1950s, the campus at Glenside accommodated about 2000 'inmates' – the largest population of people with a mental illness living in a closed community in the southern hemisphere – coming from across the state.[6]

From 1929, the site that would eventually become the Oakden Campus was established as the Northfield Mental Hospital – an additional facility for the accommodation and treatment of South Australians with a mental illness. The hospital was situated to the north of the city, across the Torrens River and some distance from the Glenside Hospital, providing better access to emerging northern communities and helping address the demand for asylum services. The campus was surrounded by pastures, vastly different to the suburban setting of 2017.

The intention was to provide asylum, given meaning through work and activity, within a standalone community. The historical record indicates that the reality was more custodial, and worse during the austerity of the intervening war years. The site became overpopulated and under-resourced as it housed increasing numbers of people of all ages with a wide range of mental health conditions, from autism to schizophrenia to dementia. Care was authoritarian. For many, home was a dormitory-style hospital ward.

Just as has occurred in other places and times, attitudes, concerns and priorities for people with mental illness fluctuated. In 1964, the name Northfield Mental Hospital was changed to the more straightforward Hillcrest Hospital. Between the 1960s and the 1980s, state funding for the hospital increased, and it arrived at a heyday – still institutional in style but with greater positivity, hope and kindness. Nurses who worked at the hospital during this period tell stories of engagement, care and pride in their work. Those who worked at Hillcrest considered themselves more innovative than their colleagues across the Torrens River at Glenside Hospital. During Hillcrest's era of optimism, there was a shift toward community-based care, and a hope of people leaving the hospital.

The hospital campus was expansive, with a stately, although austere, original building used for administration and a range of other facilities dedicated to specific populations, including accommodation for people under forensic orders, deemed not guilty of criminal acts based on having a mental illness.

In 1982, the final building to be commissioned at the Hillcrest Hospital was a new psychogeriatric unit, built as a centre for the treatment of older people with a mental illness, including people with dementia. It was built on an 'H' pattern, with a central corridor housing administrative services, flanked at four corners by wards that stretched outwards, with two- or four-bed bays, bathrooms, nurses' stations, common areas and kitchen spaces. The space was clinical and in no way homelike, but staff who worked there during the early years reported that, for a time, it was a positive service.

Services were streamed, so that people living with a mental illness, whose needs were very different to people living with dementia, were not jumbled up together. The psychogeriatric unit accommodated 123 people across four long-stay wards and one acute short-stay ward, with people living with dementia and those with mental illness each accounting for half the population. The staffing of the long-stay wards included registered and enrolled nurses specialising in mental health care. There was access to allied health practitioners, a consultant psychiatrist and a general practitioner. Two teams provided outreach to older people living in their homes in the surrounding communities. For a time, until the early 1990s, the place was a hive of activity, with day programs, colour and creativity. It may be that the service was paternalistic and institutional; however, the idea of asylum – a haven and sanctuary for people who could not find peace and safety elsewhere – informed much of the well-intentioned, albeit old-fashioned, enterprise.

In the early 1990s, Australia also began 'mainstreaming' its mental health services: a slow process of integration with the rest of its health and hospital systems. Services relocated acute mental health wards to larger general hospital campuses. The 'back-wards', housing people with chronic mental illnesses that were refractory to treatment, were progressively closed and decommissioned. Residents from these wards, which were particularly populous at the Glenside campus, moved into a range of community settings in a program entitled 'returning home'. For some, this was wonderfully successful, bringing independence, liberation and the first taste of normality after years of institutional living. Others, having only known the wards as 'home', struggled to make up the gap in function required to manage life outside the hospital.

As part of this process, Hillcrest Hospital closed in 1992. The forensic mental health service and the older persons' mental health service remained as the only two services on the campus, in a newly renamed suburb – Oakden. Other buildings were demolished or sold, setting the scene for the services to become isolated. The forensic service sat some distance from the older persons' service. It was protected by high-set security fences and locked entrances. The older persons' service sat back from the road, surrounded by car parks and tracts of grass that would later become dry and cracked with neglect. Central administrative functions, which had been part of the defunct Hillcrest Hospital, were, largely, not replaced.

The older persons' service included four long-stay wards – Makk, McLeay, Clements and Zweck – with a focus on people presenting with behavioural and psychological symptoms of dementia, blended with older people with complex, enduring mental illnesses. Howard House, the acute assessment and inpatient hospital unit, remained onsite, providing a somewhat greater level of transparency and community, supported as it was by a larger cohort of psychiatrists, registrars, allied health practitioners and administrators. The seeds of ruin might already have been planted, but for a time the slow decline continued without being noticed. Howard House, the site of my internship introduction to old age psychiatry, did not move out to join the local tertiary hospital, Lyell McEwin, until 2009 – a late recruit to the mainstreaming of services.

In 1998 a decision was made within the South Australian Department of Health to apply for accreditation of Makk and McLeay as a Commonwealth-funded nursing home. It made savvy business sense. The state could shift the funding of the service to the Commonwealth and save a lot of money. It was a tipping point in the narrative of the Oakden Campus. From that time onward, the state sought to divest itself of the budgetary burden, while the personal and clinical needs of the resident population remained unchanged. Why would any organisation invest in something of which they were trying to rid themselves? It was not possible to maintain a specialist level of service – and yet this was the facility's purpose. Oakden's deterioration was almost inevitable.

The model of care became confused and compromised. Commonwealth accreditation under the Aged Care Act was embedded with the concept of 'security of tenure', meaning a person resident in a Commonwealth-funded place of care held that place for the duration of their life. This imperative was at odds with the idea of a transitional unit that would accommodate people only for so long as they clinically needed it – which was the intention of the service. But this latter purpose was not clearly articulated, and staff provided mixed messages to families. This set the scene for the service's failure to fulfil its purpose – to provide high-level care to people with complex needs, while they required it, supporting their transition to mainstream care settings when their needs were more stable.

The staffing profile gradually reduced in numbers and skills. To manage the budgetary cost pressures, allied health practitioner roles were not backfilled when people went on leave. Positions remained vacant when staff left. The ratio of nurses and care workers delivering care on the wards dropped to close to nursing-home levels, which was all the Commonwealth accreditors required. Because of the greater complexity of the residents, the work was demanding and untenable at these staffing levels. The needs of residents were unmet.

The Commonwealth-funded wards began to run into trouble with accreditation – a sign of issues with quality and safety. Between 2001 and 2007, the Commonwealth granted accreditation for short (one- or two-year) periods. In 2007, the facility failed twenty-five of the forty-four Commonwealth aged care standards. For the first time, sanctions were imposed, and the service hit the news – briefly.

There was a flurry of activity. The service made efforts to address some of the deficits. The state government brokered a partnership with a large, successful, not-for-profit aged care provider who took over operations of services, only to withdraw from the relationship a short while later.

By 2010, the funding of maintenance or infrastructural improvements ceased, leading to the dilapidation that was found at the time of the review in 2017, at which point the service sat in isolation on Foster's Road, far removed from the more important services delivered at the network's tertiary hospital, replete with its new buildings. Bordered by tall mesh fences and surrounded by expanses of clay-cracked fields of dry grass, Oakden looked more like a prison. The underlying narrative – that this was a service without a future – had taken hold.

9

Culture, contingents and contradictions

Organisational culture is a powerful force, influencing everyone's experience in their workplace. In health and social care, the connection between culture and care is inextricable.[1] Curiously, the word 'culture' is derived from the Latin 'cultus' – meaning *care*.[2] As a review panel, it didn't take us long to conclude that Oakden's most fundamental problem was toxic culture. We knew this would be the greatest challenge to overcome. The power of culture is such that reasonable people can get caught up in it and either lose their way, giving in to the prevailing way of doing things, or lose their voice while trying to bring about change, and retreat in defeat.

Just as we listened to the families of Oakden residents, we had conversations with many staff. They had their own stories to tell. We also scoured hundreds of pages of clinical notes describing the day-to-day treatment of Oakden residents. In our interviews with staff, and in their notes written on the pages of residents' clinical records, we found underlying beliefs and attitudes, spontaneously exposed, attesting to the 'othering' that characterised the culture of the service – the 'us' of seasoned, long-established staff, and 'them' of all others: residents, families, new staff, management, and anyone else who tried to challenge the status quo. These sentiments emerged from staff seemingly without awareness, so enculturated were they in a dichotomist way of seeing the world and the people they were meant to care for.

Circumstances are rarely all one thing or the other. It is essential to acknowledge an inherent contradiction relating to the Oakden staff. It was captured by a resident's family member during their interview with the review panel.

'They weren't all bad staff,' they said. 'Some were compassionate and caring and did the very best they could with the resources they had.'

The problem was that the voices of these caring staff were hardly heard against the rampant culture of institutional dehumanisation.

❖❖❖

'We want the old psych ward days back,' said one of the nurses to the review panel. 'That was when it worked.'

'The staff are doing the same things they did in the back-wards at the old Glenside hospital twenty-five years ago,' another staff member explained.

We came to understand what this meant, as we heard and read about the antiquated asylum style of treatment.

'Locking their doors is about limit-setting,' a nurse told us, when explaining the practice of locking residents out of their own rooms, restricting them from freely accessing private and personal space. The terminology 'limit-setting' smacked of a nineteenth-century boarding school.

We read about residents being 'nursed in a low-stimulus environment'. We came to understand this was a euphemism for seclusion – keeping residents isolated in spaces they could not get out of.

'As long as there's a danger to self and others, there's a shade of grey,' a nurse stated in explaining the rationale for the frequent use of restraint. 'You need to be able to do a restraint at the drop of a hat,' they said, indifferent toward the practice of strapping someone into a chair.

There weren't enough staff to respond to residents if they were agitated or fell over, without leaving others unattended. To manage this, residents were restrained into seats or reclined in princess chairs, unable to get out. The use of restraints was coupled with liberal use of psychotropic medications, as a means of managing the frustration and consequent agitation of the residents due to their immobilisation.

In 2016 there were approximately 3000 documented incidents of mechanical restraint at the Oakden Campus. Benchmarking indicated that this was more than the total number of restraints used in adult mental health services across the rest of Australia during the same period.[3] We became aware that there were other, undocumented, incidents of restraint and seclusion – like Bob Spriggs experienced. The use of these restrictive practices was so habitual and normalised that many staff didn't consider it necessary to report them. They were perceived as the only way to cope.

We heard about some residents having six or seven staff simultaneously attend to personal hygiene. We struggled to imagine what made this necessary, let alone consider the trauma it would cause.

We were told about the 'Clements' morning line-up'. Residents of the Clements ward were regimented to get out of bed at 7:30 am, whether it suited them or not. Breakfast was not until 8 am, so residents were lined up outside their rooms, in a long corridor, until being marched around to the large common room that served as a living, dining, sitting and everything space. The residents then began their long day of unscheduled inactivity.

We were told about weekend staff bringing laptops and movies to entertain themselves during their twelve-hour shifts, rather than providing care for the residents.

The loss of humanity and hope was palpable.

'These people,' said one senior nurse, with disdain, 'can't get any better.' They rationalised that the loss of allied health clinicians did not matter, as the residents of Oakden could not benefit from such input. 'We don't need an occupational therapist,' the nurse said. 'These people can't be rehabilitated.'

Another nurse likened the residents of Oakden to wild animals in a circus. With relish, they described themselves as a 'ringmaster' who 'had the knack', adding: 'You can't teach that!'

Still another nurse stated, 'I just can't find anything good about these people.'

As we searched the clinical records, there was limited evidence of staff connecting residents' behaviours with their changed capacity and challenges communicating hunger, thirst, pain, anxiety or loneliness. Instead, we found a predominance of pejorative and derisive language.

We found descriptors of residents being 'uncooperative', 'non-compliant', 'aggressive', 'intrusive', 'abusive toward staff' and 'assaultive'. Residents 'refused' and 'resisted' when staff were attending to task lists. They were described as being 'behavioural' and 'difficult', implying that they were somehow being deliberately oppositional, creating challenging conditions for the staff.

Language is at the heart of culture. The way we think, write and speak about people is crucial. Words can create self-fulfilling expectations around what people will be like and how they will behave. At Oakden, a dehumanised view of residents, reinforced through language, perpetuated a culture of dehumanising treatment. The treatment of residents compounded their behaviours, which expressed unmet needs and deep discontent – further 'proving' that the staff's perceptions were correct: the residents were the problem.

The clinical records at Oakden were particularly notable for this use of language, but there are elements of this cultural phenomenon in many healthcare settings. It is interesting to wonder how simple changes – like switching 'refuse' to 'decline' or 'making their own choice', for instance – might have shifted how residents were *seen* and how staff *felt* about their work.[4]

Oakden's identity of neglect and impoverishment was inculcated at a cultural level. Just as residents' family members had done, the staff spoke of the dictum *'there is no money'*. We were told of basic clinical equipment, like blood pressure cuffs, not being replaced and staff being told to make do.

'Stop asking for things you're not going to get,' one staff member reported being told.

The loss of humanity extended to the identity of the staff

themselves. They were aware of their place as the 'others' of the health system. There was deep distrust of the distant executives, whom the staff believed knew nothing of their lives. They believed themselves to be misunderstood and disliked.

'We're a backwater,' a staff member told the panel.

'We're a team of misfits,' said another, capturing the intrinsic identity of the service.

'They've forgotten us and don't care,' concluded another.

❖ ❖ ❖

We spoke with the executives, whom the staff considered to be distant and unconcerned, who were responsible for Oakden when the story first broke in early 2017. We recognised that they represented the cumulation of a line of predecessors. Executives personify cultures of belief, attitude and practice as much as anyone at the frontline. Their decisions have far-reaching effects, filtering throughout an organisation. Decisions – such as the withdrawal of allied health staff or the setting of nursing hours per resident similar to typical residential aged care facilities, despite the work being much more demanding – were the result of budget constraints. Distance protected the executives from awareness of the impact on the people at the end of these decisions, both staff and residents.

There were stories of attempts made by middle managers to cobble together temporary social work, occupational therapy and psychology positions, none of which lasted. By the end of 2016, a part-time dietician was the only allied health practitioner remaining. There was a cavernous gap between the executives' understanding of the nature of the work, the resources required, and what was approved and delivered. We found the general executive response was ignorance of what was going on and reliance on middle management to address issues.

There was a range of reasons that might account for the fact that executives did not know what was going on. They were busy. Very busy. There were budgetary pressures to manage in a landscape of fiscal limitation. They were under constant pressure from their bosses in the Department of Health. There were continual rounds of briefings and reports – mostly concerned with the bottom line and never the forgotten older people at Oakden, who lived beyond the bottom line.

The executives did not visit Oakden. They had not spoken with the residents or their families. If the service had been closed and the budget redirected, they would likely have been relieved, and none the wiser about what was really happening.

The executives also carried the constant burden of systems 'flow', informed by preeminent, mandated key performance indicators regarding how much time a person spends in an emergency department. The problems associated with people experiencing waits in overrun emergency departments are recognised globally. The flow-on effect of this is the need to move people through acute hospital stays efficiently, keeping bed occupancy such that there is always the ability to admit someone presenting to the emergency department to the right place, at the right time, the first time.

Trouble with 'flow' occurs when parts of the system are imbalanced and cannot respond to demand. When it comes to an ageing population, acute health services do not exist in isolation from aged care services, and if these sectors are not working in concert with each other – which is often the case – bottlenecks and breakdowns occur. The same applies to all sorts of people with complex problems who require more sophisticated support to find pathways for recovery. Such people can easily become stranded and be the source of 'flow issues'. It's easy for a culture of blame to develop around this.

One of the reasons Oakden continued for so long without challenge was because it provided a release valve for system flow issues. It was not that the executives who perpetuated this prioritisation of flow were inherently uncaring; it was that the pressured *mechanics* of system flow screamed more loudly than the human stories that occurred downstream from decision-making.

To illustrate this, a year before the Oakden story broke, one of the network executives directed that a man in his fifties – Jeff – who lived with chronic, treatment-resistant schizophrenia, should be admitted to Oakden. Jeff had become 'stranded' in an acute adult mental health service. No one could identify a viable management plan to support his recovery and accommodation, and there was increasing pressure for him to move 'somewhere more appropriate' – whatever this undefined term meant. Without understanding his needs or considering the appropriateness of placing him where most residents had dementia, Jeff was sent to Oakden so he would no longer be 'blocking a bed'.

In the months following his admission, Jeff's mental state deteriorated. He was kept in isolation much of the time because of his incompatibility with the other residents. Staff were afraid of him as he lumbered menacingly around his corner of the ward, muttering an incomprehensible monologue. His quality of life was appalling. He appeared unhappy and irritable. He eventually pushed another (much older) resident over, causing him a subdural haematoma – a bleed into his brain.

Much later, after the Oakden Report, as the closure of the campus was being navigated and reform was underway, Jeff was readmitted to the acute adult mental health service so he could have a treatment trial with clozapine, the best available (albeit high-risk) medical treatment for schizophrenia.

He was transformed. He appeared clear-eyed, calm and was able to have a coherent conversation. A short while later, he transitioned out of state-run mental health services and found a new home with a community-based, compassionate, non-government, not-for-profit support team. This transition could have occurred eighteen months earlier but had been intercepted by a disconnected executive decision, reflecting short-sighted visibility of immediate efficiency and flow rather than understanding the person and their situation.

❖ ❖ ❖

What happened to the middle managers responsible for Oakden – the Medical Director, Nursing Director and Service Manager – was particularly disturbing. They were caught, aware that the service was not fit for purpose but unable or unprepared to speak up. It seemed they felt disempowered, perceiving an adversarial relationship with the executives, and believing that they were unsupported. At the same time, they managed upwards, trying in vain to make things work by complying with budgetary constraints, which could only be done by delivering a sub-standard service. It was a catch-22. The review panel came to understand that these middle managers were aware they were sitting on a simmering calamity that would one day erupt into a scandal – but seemed unable to do anything about it.

The review heard that workplace incidents, performance and staff conduct problems were inadequately addressed. After the Oakden Report, when thousands of documents were subpoenaed by the Independent Commissioner Against Corruption, a drawer of files regarding incidents of misconduct was found in one of the middle managers' offices, with no evidence that any of them had been actioned. The result of this approach to management was the fostering of a belief that some staff were untouchable, while others, hoping to do the right thing, felt discouraged and vulnerable.

We learnt that a nursing leader, who was trying earnestly to bring about positive change, witnessed misconduct toward a resident by a staff member. He was advised by one of the middle managers not to report the incident to the Nurses Board, despite there being a clear justification for doing so. Aware that no other action had been taken, the nursing leader went ahead and reported the incident, convinced that this was the right thing to do – but with trepidation regarding the possibility of retribution for speaking up.

There was a practice of sending poor-performing staff from elsewhere across mental health services to work at Oakden, as if it was some type of purgatory. This was used as a means of shifting problems from elsewhere and avoiding having to diligently support workforce improvement. We were told about one poorly performing staff member from another site who was sent to Oakden on a 'performance improvement plan', with the instruction to 'manage him out' quietly added as an aside to the receiving supervisor at Oakden.

The transferred staff member allegedly sat in an office for the duration of the secondment with very few duties and no education to support their growth. The review heard of staff who were recruited from overseas to work in mental health services, and who were discovered to have gaps in their qualifications. They were placed at Oakden.

The review panel was told that, at times of Commonwealth aged care accreditation, 'problem' staff were sent home before assessors arrived at the building – including both those who might stand out to assessors as deficient, and those who were suspiciously viewed as potential whistleblowers on the realities of life at Oakden. Better quality staff were 'borrowed' from other services to get through accreditation and then returned to their substantive positions once assessments were complete.[5]

We found a lack of honesty in the way documentation was managed during aged care accreditation. Two separate sets of notes were maintained for the same resident. There were the 'hospital notes', containing more comprehensive clinical information, and 'aged care notes' relating only to issues of aged care accreditation. The 'aged care notes' were made available to Commonwealth assessors, while the 'hospital notes' were shelved, concealing critical information. The practice was inefficient, unsafe, and raised a red flag regarding culture and governance. Why keep things secret?

The review panel heard about the efforts of some staff to escalate their concerns to these middle managers and the executives, attempting to flag risks. The dwindling presence of allied health practitioners, the high rates of seclusion and restraint, reports of bullying and misconduct among staff were all raised as problems. Many emails remained unanswered.

In 2014, a senior consultant psychiatrist, acting briefly as the Clinical Director, placed the service on the organisational risk register. It stayed there for a while, before being removed by agreement between the middle managers and the executives with the justification that the risk had been 'resolved'. Nothing had been done. Nothing had changed.

There was a trail of hopeful clinicians who had taken jobs at Oakden over numerous years, believing they would be listened to when speaking up. Very few lasted long. Confronted by daily toxicity and meeting resistance to change from those responsible for governance, these clinicians retreated and left. Some later spoke out publicly about their experiences.[6] Frustration and hopelessness were common themes.

One nurse reported how, when she started working at Oakden, she couldn't understand why there was no toilet paper in the bathrooms.

'We put everyone in continence pads when they arrive,' she was told by a long-standing staff member. 'It's much easier for us to manage – and the toilet paper was blocking the pipes.'

The new nurse felt horrified, viewing such a strategy as restrictive and lacking in dignity. She proposed a research project that promoted continence by encouraging residents to get back to using the toilet – complete with toilet paper. By weighing continence pads – which got lighter – she proved the strategy worked. There was increased independent use of the toilets, and decreased use of continence aids – both supporting dignity and saving money – with no blocked toilets.

Resistance to the project was such that the nurse eventually moved on, feeling frustrated by the Oakden culture. Things returned to baseline.

❖❖❖

Reflecting on the stories told by executives and managers, the review panel was struck by the failure to take responsibility. This observation was summarised in the Report:

> It had become a situation of people taking aim at others they perceived to be responsible. The result had been a circular firing squad with no one working to solve the problem. Many have stood by, incurious and disinterested, and watched it happen.

To her credit, when Jackie Hanson, CEO of the health network, sat before the Senate select committee, established in 2017 to explore further the question of who was responsible for the failures at Oakden, she had the fortitude to say: 'The buck stopped with me.'

There was no blame shifting, no effort to mitigate responsibility by claiming ignorance. By this time, Jackie had worked out that ignorance was not a valid excuse, and she was courageous enough to acknowledge it. Not everyone had discovered this. Remarkably, during the review, only one senior staff member acknowledged that they had failed to do their job.

When the Independent Commissioner Against Corruption, Bruce Lander QC, released his report in 2018, the three primary middle managers at Oakden were found guilty of maladministration.[7] The organisation was found guilty, but no single executive, nor any member of the government, was directly called to account.

The onus was on the organisation to take ownership of the failures wholly and voluntarily – and what might be learnt from them. Without current and future leadership taking responsibility, there is a risk of diluting the narrative regarding the higher-level organisational failings at Oakden. It's worth contemplating the potential implications of this in terms of culture reform. If there is not heartfelt change at the highest level within an organisation, bridging the gap of disconnection, where will the sustainable support for frontline culture change come from?

❖ ❖ ❖

What struck us most about the culture at Oakden, as we delved into the experiences of the people who worked there, was the impact of isolation and neglect in creating a social environment all of its own. It was uncannily reminiscent of the altered morality and 'groupthink' described in William Golding's fictional account of British boys stranded on an Island in his 1954 book, *Lord of the Flies*.[8]

There is a colloquial idea of the 'nursing mafia' – a group of nurses who hold sway over others within a health service, well known for 'eating their own' and inducing fear in younger, less experienced nurses. In the microcosm at Oakden there was a dominant culture characterised by bullying, intimidation and pressure to conform.

Culture, contingents and contradictions

Within this culture, there were power players who took up unofficial leadership of the service as if it was a cause, their faces set against the outside world in opposition. Prominent among these was a nurse commonly referred to as 'Teflon'.

Teflon was an older nurse, carved out in the institutional model. He was known as 'Teflon' because he had been the subject of numerous suspensions and investigations following allegations of misconduct, none of which had stuck. The charges against him unproven, he repeatedly returned to the workplace jubilant at his victory over impotent management. For those in leadership, 'Teflon' was a term of derision. For Teflon and his allies, it was a provocative commendation. One staff member sincerely informed the review that Teflon was the 'grandmaster' of the service.

Teflon would take it upon himself on each of his shifts to go 'rounding'. He would walk around each of the wards, visible and present. He would place a hand on a shoulder, letting his people know that he was there for them. On days when he did not work, he would take dinner and snacks in for the staff, to fill their stomachs and warm their souls. They were *his* wards, and he spoke of them in these terms. Superficially, he was the epitome of altruistic service.

The review was told a story by one of the visiting geriatricians. This extremely competent young woman had attended Oakden regularly, providing, through time-limited visits, the best supportive advice she could. On one occasion she had reviewed one of the residents and was standing at the medication trolley, looking at a chart and amending an order.

'Get away from my medication charts, girlie!' Teflon yelled across the room, waving his arms at her. It was a misaligned declamation that captured Teflon's sense of ownership and a festering culture of disrespect.

So embedded was the culture of separatism and resistance that a special language developed to communicate the presence of management or medical staff. The review heard how, when a senior staff member stepped onto one of the wards, a whispered 'boss-on-floor' would spread from one end of the ward to the other, twisting around corners and reaching everyone with the warning to be on their best behaviour. This strategy was so well oiled that the medical officer and one of the nursing leads, valiantly trying to advocate for change, took to wearing softer shoes and unlocking doors silently, to avoid announcing their arrival.

To suggest that Teflon's style of treatment was paternalistic would be an understatement. He referred to himself as 'Uncle'.

'Come on,' he would whisper into the ear of a distressed resident, holding them firmly. 'It's Uncle here; you *behave* yourself.'

The review learnt of incidents in which he had used undue force in physically handling residents. He was witnessed pushing a person who did not want to sit down into a chair, punching the air afterwards in a victory salute, and laughing with a colleague as he celebrated his ascendency over the recalcitrant resident.

'Job well done,' he stated in his explanation of this incident, when asked about it in the review.

There were many such allegations. There was a report that Teflon pushed a resident's fingers between a chair and a table and held them there. There was alleged pushing and shoving, and speaking to residents coercively and with condescension, rather than kindness and collaboration. He represented a prison-like hierarchy in which the residents were required to comply, and staff needed to toe the line with power-broking wardens. Teflon and the nursing 'mafia' made it impossible for dissenting staff to feel they had somewhere they could go with their concerns, fearful of recriminations for speaking up.

Teflon first spoke to the review panel during a group session. He had charisma. The other panel members and I were already seated, with plenty of space for the staff to gather comfortably around a large conference table. Bizarrely, Teflon smacked his lips, came around to where I was sitting and, without introducing himself, pulled up a chair so close to mine that we were physically touching. He sat down theatrically. Then he said, with pointed emphasis, 'Well, *someone's* uncomfortable, aren't they?' He passed a sidelong squint in my direction.

To be sure, this behaviour did make me uncomfortable, but I greeted him, introduced myself and – despite having worked out who he was, given the stories we had already heard – asked him who he was. In loud, staccato letters he spelled out his name for me, surname first, and then repeated it, almost rolling his consonants for dramatic effect. Perhaps thinking better of his conduct, he backed down somewhat and pulled his chair away from mine to a more socially appropriate distance. Throughout the session the other staff said little, but dutifully agreed while Teflon waxed eloquently.

You do not need to be a psychiatrist to work out that there was some pathological behaviour here. This one interaction provided insight into Teflon as an individual, but it also opened a window on the world within Oakden, where a larger-than-life, controlling personality like Teflon could wreak havoc on the landscape of safe working relationships. Unchecked and magnified by the countless number of staff who had lost their way, a culture of contempt had permeated the service. One might wonder what role Oakden played in meeting Teflon's psychological needs. He found identity, power, and a potent sense of agency on his wards.

Shortly before the release of the Oakden Report, the organisation closed in on the allegations surrounding Teflon and suspended him again. He was in his seventies, and he died suddenly before completion of this final investigation. His family and friends mourned; police interviews with witnesses continued.

When I heard about Teflon's death, I felt conflicted, struggling with the inclination to think of him as an 'all-bad' person. Yet, as misguided as Teflon was, this was not the case. I imagined how things would've looked if he'd let go of his overattachment to the service at Oakden years earlier, rather than drawing his identity from his role, manufactured in the isolated community. He might have enjoyed more time with his family or redirected his energy into different work. Perhaps he was another victim of the broad system failure that allowed such conditions to prosper, fostering the errant attachments and behaviours of people like him. Making sense of Teflon's narrative requires us to look for the humanity in his story as much as we might do for someone who meets with our approval.

❖❖❖

At the end of this difficult chapter in the Oakden story, it's important to recall that, while there was a dominant toxic culture at Oakden, there were also gems of kindness, commitment and care hidden away among the staff. We later saw these staff emerging as champions in our reinvented service at Northgate House, able to deliver the care they aspired to. It is necessary to confront the disturbing truth and learn from what went wrong in the culture of the Oakden workforce, and to consider how this might have relevance in other settings, recognising that staff at all levels in an organisation contribute to culture – from the C-suite to the coalface. At the same time, it is valuable to recognise that seeds of hope and humanity were tucked away in decent people who hung on, eager for change and committed to serving the people in their care. They were quietly unsung heroes, eclipsed by the dysfunction, but still doing their best while they waited for things to turn around. The presence of these contingents creates the contradiction of the Oakden staff stories.

10

A steep and strenuous climb

The Oakden Report was released in April 2017. It outlined disturbing findings and made six key recommendations: the need for a model of care describing new services; design and development of purpose-built environments; nurturing of quality staff; provision of good governance; removal of restrictive practices like restraint; and the all-important work of culture reform, offering transformation.

Amid the political and public pandemonium that followed, there was a vacuum in the clinical leadership of the Older Persons' Mental Health Service. A highly challenging job desperately needed doing. Executives and consultants were stepping in, both responding to and exacerbating a climate of extreme reactivity. I received a call from the Director of Mental Health Services, asking me if I'd come and help.

Aaron Groves saw potential pitfalls ahead. 'Don't do it,' he advised.

He could (correctly) see the potential for a Royal Commission and was uncertain how the South Australian Government and Department of Health would manage their responses. His concern was that I might be made a scapegoat for failure in a system where diligent follow-through could not be relied upon.

Steven Garber's words regarding vocation are relevant here. When he posed the question, 'Why get involved?', he responded:

It is one thing to know about messes, but it is something else altogether to step into a mess. It is one thing to know about things being wrong, but it's something else altogether to decide that I am responsible to make it right.[1]

For better or worse, I believed this was a chance to make a difference in something important. So, less than a month after the release of the report, I walked onsite at Oakden again, this time with the momentous responsibility of unravelling the contents of the Pandora's box of which I had a hand in opening.

My first moments did not go well. With a sense of grave importance, I opened the front door, infamously positioned next to the plant room. I stepped inside onto the shiny, hard vinyl, which only moments earlier had been mopped (reflecting newly enforced efforts to present the building as sparkling clean). My feet swiftly left the floor, flying forwards into the air while the rest of my body slammed backwards onto the ground. I was winded and wounded – albeit the damage was mostly to my ego. I sincerely hoped this was not a portent of what was about to happen to my life and career.

A couple of staff heard the commotion and came to my aid as I struggled off the floor, humiliated and awkward.

'Hello, I'm the new Head of Unit,' I announced, painfully aware of the inauspiciousness of my arrival.

The incident stays with me as a symbolic reminder of the value of deconstructing the power differentials that prevent us being real with each other in health services – and elsewhere. Not that I would ever wish a spectacular fall on anyone else. There are better ways to level the field.

There had been an ironic pendulum swing by the time the Oakden Report was published. Having been a victim of abject neglect and lack of interest, Oakden became the focus of organisational, political and public attention. The decision had already been taken, prior to me commencing, that Oakden was too far gone and would close. It was to be replaced by a much smaller, interim service in two buildings, yet to be refurbished, rented from the Department of Human Services, in the neighbouring suburb of Northgate.

A steep and strenuous climb

Where before there had been a narrative of 'no money for that', suddenly there was great agility in mobilising resources. Jackie Hanson told me how, early on, while the review was still underway, she had informed her bosses in the department that if she were going to fix what had happened, she would need to do it properly – which would mean spending whatever it cost. Resources were rapidly pulled from other sites across the health network – staff from all disciplines, budget for renovations, educational resources – some of which were thrown around willy-nilly. Infrastructure repairs at Oakden, for instance, were undertaken precipitously, despite there being awareness that the service would be closing. Teams from other services looked on with mixed emotions: judgement of the service for being so deplorable; relief that they were not so deficient themselves; resentment that Oakden was the centre of attention and receiving rapid reallocation of support, which was perceived to compromise other areas.

I was, of course, grateful for the availability of resources. If I needed something, I seemed to be able to get it – for a while, at least. But the initial period of agility was not underpinned by clear thinking on sustainability. I wondered what would happen once the dust settled, and everyone moved on to the next big issue. It wasn't long before there were mutterings from the state treasury about the reallocation of budget after the closure of Oakden. I earnestly argued that, for the same cost that had previously run a more extensive service of inferior quality, I could develop a smaller service of very high quality. The need to have an articulated vision and model of care to inform the dimensions and future direction of our services became increasingly important.

The pendulum also swung from a lack of governance to extreme levels of scrutiny and control. Everything was reported. Protocols were established that included reporting every incident to the state Minister for Mental Health. Ironic, given that her pre-emptive visit never happened. Police reports were filed frequently. These were done in person. Online reports to the health practitioner registration agency and the Independent Commissioner Against Corruption became almost daily occurrences for a time.

Meetings were set up to create visibility over everything. Each working day commenced as early as 7 am with a 'war room' meeting, involving all the executives and the immediate Oakden response team. A group of us worked continuously, easily double time, with emails often being sent around at 2 or 3 am. It was intense and insane – and certainly not sustainable.

The Commonwealth Aged Care Quality Agency, which had delivered a three-year accreditation to Oakden in late 2016, came back in February 2017, after news stories emerged in the media but before the release of the report. Caught out and embarrassed by the failures in their accreditation processes, they declared Oakden to be the worst facility they had ever seen, immediately issuing sanctions that required profound remedial action.

As a further irony, the failure of the Quality Agency concerning the accreditation of Oakden became the focus of a review commissioned by Ken Wyatt AM, MP, then federal Minister for Senior Australians and Aged Care, leading to substantial changes in the structure and function of the agency itself – with a profound impact across the entire aged care sector.[2] Sanctions were delivered thick and fast to aged care providers across the country. It seemed that from the perspective of the Agency – which subsequently became the Aged Care Quality and Safety Commission – these actions were considered duly diligent in setting the standard. From the standpoint of providers, it felt like a new era of punitive action had begun, out of step with the landscape of limited resources and capability throughout the sector, in which issues could not be resolved within the timeframes expected. Simply telling providers that they were not good enough did not solve the problems.

Back at Oakden, the assessors from the Commonwealth came every day. They would arrive at unannounced times, including weekends and evenings, and had access to every aspect of the service operations. We were working extremely hard to address the many problems and provide better care. But it became apparent that, no matter what we did, there would be an outcome of being deemed beyond repair.

Oakden and the Northern Adelaide Local Health Network were to be a cautionary tale – an example to all who might not take the issues of quality and safety seriously in the future. The pendulum had swung in the other direction and approved aged care provider status was withdrawn.

Before I arrived at Oakden, I had some residual hope that we could salvage the service and, refurbished, have it rise like a phoenix, but it took only a short time for me to agree that the only option was complete closure. The standards of care, the service culture, and the extreme reactivity surrounding the service in the organisational, political and public landscape made this inevitable. I quickly realised that the decision to move to the much smaller service at Northgate, allowing radical change, was the best opportunity for reinvention. The most significant problem, at this time of swinging pendulums, was the overarching punitive tone of interactions between agencies, levels of the organisation and individuals.

❖❖❖

Organisational change theorist Ed Schein described motivation to learn and change as the consequence of several conditions. Schein argued that unless people feel *safe* enough to learn, they can be told all manner of things without hearing them. If people do not feel safe, suggestions that there are areas for growth will be defended against. People will not acknowledge their need for change or be motivated to act on it. Schein referred to the conditions required for learning and growth as 'psychological safety'.[3]

Amy Edmondson is a leading researcher and writer on psychological safety. She wrote:

> *Psychological safety describes a belief that neither the formal nor informal consequences of interpersonal risks, like asking for help or admitting a failure, will be punitive. In psychologically safe environments, people believe that if they make a mistake or ask for help, others will not react badly. Instead, candor is both allowed*

and expected. Psychological safety exists when people feel their workplace is an environment where they can speak up, offer ideas and ask questions without fear of being punished or embarrassed.

Fear works in opposition to psychological safety and inhibits learning. Edmondson has pointed out that hierarchy, handled poorly, creates anxiety and reduces psychological safety. When people are afraid of getting in trouble from those higher-up, they lose access to memory and information processing, impairing problem-solving and creativity.[4]

❖ ❖ ❖

In the first days and months after taking up the role at Oakden, I was exposed first-hand to a hierarchical and punitive approach that sought blame and told people how bad they were. It was a potent impediment to positive growth. Change was forced upon people, and compliance was demanded. To a point, it is understandable that this occurred but, in retrospect, I do not doubt that the result was further trauma and damage to many of the staff involved, rather than the development of a service where change starts with the heart. For some staff, I contributed to this experience of punitive action. Becoming immersed in this situation was the start of my process of learning, in which the ideas of psychological safety and the deconstruction of hierarchies became increasingly important. What I learnt ultimately changed my life – but at the beginning it was painful.

Two consultants were brought from interstate to help with the reform efforts. They were nurses who, approaching the end of their careers, had been elevated to peripatetic experts in aged care, advising struggling services.

On my first day, having recovered from my spectacular fall, I met the senior consultant.

'Who are you?' she demanded.

'I'm the new Head of Unit …' I began.

'Well, you'll need to be speaking with *me*, then, won't you,' she interrupted.

She carried an air of authority that defied questioning. She appeared confident that she had the backing of the Commonwealth in her dire assessment of the service strewn around her, and she held little back.

The fact was, she did have a thorough knowledge of the aged care sector. She was correct in her judgement of the service at Oakden. The problem was that team members experienced her manner as harsh – vicious, even – when they were trying hard to change things. The consultant's vitriol was met with angst and animus. Staff were left either in tears or enraged following interactions with her. Nothing positive came from these encounters.

Both consultants were unceremoniously (and disrespectfully) referred to, by all and sundry, without charity – although never when they were around.

'Those *awful* women …' I heard people say.

There was a collective sigh of relief when both consultants went back home. I suspect they had formed the view that we were a lost cause. I had much to learn regarding the building of psychological safety. Still, these two consultants exemplified the adage that 'you catch more flies with honey than vinegar'. Had they been more mindful of this, they may not have missed the opportunity to make a positive difference.

❖❖❖

The punitive tone was not limited to those working within the organisation. Interactions with the various industrial bodies were also contentious. The unions expressed outrage that Oakden had occurred but frequently argued over the reform process.

The Oakden Report recommended ceasing twelve-hour shifts for nurses in this highly exhausting area of practice. The professional arm of the nurses' union agreed that this was appropriate, but the industrial arm of the union fought hard – representing paid-up members who were opposed to change – and slowed progress.

I found it bizarre that I was dragged in to attend the industrial commission to resolve a dispute over office space, when there were so many more important issues to address. I was infuriated one day to find a nurses' union representative in one of the medication rooms, distracting staff while they were trying to prepare a medication order for a resident – seemingly unconcerned that this increased the risk of an error that could cause harm. I was incensed when a union representative alleged that our leadership team was motivated by self-interest rather than the real-world reform of our service. We needed partners in change – not opponents.

❖ ❖ ❖

Having acknowledged a reactive and punitive organisational climate, it's also important to be clear that there were real deficits and failures that required a decisive response. The care delivered by some staff was substandard and needed to be addressed. Educational, practice and HR challenges were real.

One day, very early in the change process, I was in McLeay House. An older woman, who had lost her ability to communicate verbally, and had been lying back in a princess chair, was trying to sit up and get out of the chair. A staff member walked past her on the way to do another task and perfunctorily compelled her back into the chair by placing his hand on her forehead, pushing and unbalancing her. Here was an example of the dehumanised behaviour that had become part of business as usual. It was necessary to make it clear that this was not okay.

❖ ❖ ❖

Alongside the specific corrective processes with individual staff, there were efforts to upskill and educate. Programs on medication safety, person-centred care, reducing restraint, and responding to behavioural and psychological symptoms of dementia were rolled out rapid-fire.

Recruitment of new staff commenced – to the extent that interim budgets allowed – and the number of staff on the floor increased. Senior nursing staff, borrowed from elsewhere in the network, provided support through each shift. We had a couple of medical officers and, as efforts progressed, we added an occupational therapist and physiotherapist. These people became the nucleus of our developing team.

These changes provided benefits, but I was increasingly aware that profound, service-wide, heartfelt transformation at a cultural level was required, and this could not be expected to occur quickly. Lasting change takes time.

The task of dealing with so much conflict, so many people's emotions, and the operational workload that comes with managing a national scandal was enormous. No one could do it alone. At the nucleus of the enterprise was a team who worked to close the Oakden Campus, open the fledgling service at Northgate House, and articulate a plan for new services.

In addition to myself, there was Kurt, the executive lead, borrowed from the Aboriginal Health Service to supervise the operations. There was also Kate, who came in as a project officer, seconded from the Patient Safety and Quality Unit, first looking after paperwork relating to Commonwealth accreditation and, later, when aged care accreditation was gone forever, providing support for the planning of future services. In the slender breaks she allowed herself when needing to decompress, Kate could knit thread that looked like spider's web on the tiniest needles I'd ever seen. It was a stressful time for all of us, made memorable through mateship.

One of our first tasks was to transition about fifty people from the Oakden Campus into aged care placements within a matter of weeks. Remembering that dementia is not static, but rather a progressive condition, a person's care needs can change over time. For many of the people who lived at Oakden, the complex symptoms that resulted in them being admitted were no longer prominent, and they could find new, permanent homes with quality aged care providers.

With so much public attention and such a dreadful reputation, this was no easy feat. I knew we needed exceptional social workers with tenacious negotiation skills. I called on two remarkable people, Jacqui and Claire, with whom I had worked before and who I knew would be able to do the job, as well as bring some hope and humour. One of my psychiatry colleagues, Luiza, and a local geriatrician, came and diligently reassessed every person living at Oakden, to work out who needed continuing specialist care and who didn't.

Over two months of intense work, Jacqui and Claire managed to secure placements for most of the residents. Some like-minded colleagues from within the aged care industry supported us. A couple of service providers broke the mould of criticism and offered help.

'We sent people there,' said one, 'perhaps we should be prepared to take them back.'

But not all were supportive. During a meeting with several providers, I found myself on the back foot, assertively challenged about the level of state government support for local aged care providers in managing this population of older people. This was way beyond my delegation – a question for the minister – and I could not provide a reasonable response. It was an insight into the degree to which aged care providers felt abandoned by the government and inadequately supported. Little did I know how much more pressure they would encounter once the Oakden-triggered Royal Commission commenced.

Nonetheless, we forged partnerships with several providers and successfully transitioned most residents into permanent homes. Moving a person with dementia from one environment to another is never ideal. Although disruptive, it is sometimes necessary. Getting used to new places, people and routines can be hard for a person with dementia, and it shouldn't be surprising if anxiety, stress and irritability increase during a time of transition (the fact is, change can be hard for anyone, with or without dementia). But, with extra support, transitions can be successfully navigated, and the person with dementia can settle into their new home comfortably.

We set up a 'wrap-around' system, with financial support for the providers to increase the level of personal care for transitioned residents through an early adjustment period. We organised follow-up care from local community older persons' mental health services. We set up packages of increased care through non-government agencies to provide personally engaging activity for these residents. Combined with frequent checking in with the facilities, the enterprise was highly successful and, despite a couple of near misses, none of the transitioned residents presented ever again to acute hospital services needing specialist mental health or dementia care. There are some clues in this strategy regarding how care might best be provided in all aged and social care settings – recognising that there would be a cost to achieve this.

❖ ❖ ❖

While all this was going on, we waited for the facility in Northgate to become available. In the context of uncharitable media reporting, and perhaps hoping to appear assertive and in control, the Minister for Mental Health took it upon herself to issue a directive, giving us five days to complete the renovation. A remarkably capable logistician called Mandy had been brought in to manage the renovation. Despite her exceptional organisational ability, not even Mandy could deliver within such a timeframe. We pushed back against the impossible, and the minister conceded to three weeks for the renovation, a challenge we achieved to the day.

Such a short timeline meant there was little opportunity to involve the people who would use the facility in its design, nor space for reflection on how the environment would support dignified care. Yet we earnestly hoped that openness, light, the flow of movement and easy access to the outside would change the lives of residents who were used to being cooped up in poorly lit interiors at Oakden. There were stoushes with infection control officers over soft furnishings and the use of carpet. I advocated strongly for the most homelike environment we could provide.

'You can't have carpet,' said the infection control team from the acute hospital. 'You'll never keep it clean and the whole place will smell.'

I cited evidence regarding the reduced rate of injury from people falling over in carpeted areas and pointed out that we wanted to dampen sound.[5] I argued that we could clean and replace carpet tiles if necessary. We were given carpets and never regretted it.

There was limited space in the unit and nowhere for traditional nurses' stations – usually benched areas keeping 'patients' separated from the nurses who provide them care, often with glass screens for further separation and security. We embraced the opportunity to promote a model optimising engagement between staff and the people residing in the unit. Without nurses' stations, staff could not retreat to work on computers behind desks. Instead, we purchased movable workstations-on-wheels so staff could keep up with documentation while remaining present and increasing interaction with people throughout the unit. At first, the idea appeared unpalatable to nurses familiar with traditional healthcare environments – but it worked.

We moved into the new unit in June 2017. The early days encouraged optimism and hope of change, while presenting repeated challenges that reflected a workforce carrying the impact of trauma. At that stage, approximately seventy per cent of the staff had worked at Oakden; the rest were drawn from casual and agency staff.

On the first day we moved in there was chaos. Both residents and staff were disrupted and out of place. One resident, a man called John, with younger-onset dementia, became distressed and agitated. The best way he had to manage his anxiety was to physically defend himself from anyone who came near him. Had he been given time and space, he may have been able to de-escalate. A large, athletic male nurse from the casual pool was on shift. He was a friendly and decent nurse, but not experienced in this type of situation. His efforts to compel compliance from John only made things worse. He ended up trying to control John's behaviour by throwing a towel over his head as a handler might do to manage a wild animal. Another staff member eventually stepped in and took control, and thankfully John calmed down.

Within days of moving in, we saw changes in many of the residents. They were visibly calmer, exploring the gardens, instead of being restricted indoors as had been the case at Oakden. Anthony, our gifted and determined physiotherapist, managed to get residents back up walking instead of being confined to chairs. Residents who had not spoken for a long time started to communicate again. We started to see the potential for the re-enablement of people with dementia who had been written off as incapable of recovery. We had already ceased the use of mechanical restraints, such as lap belts, before leaving Oakden, and the team were increasingly proud of not having these devices at Northgate House.

I was already committed to the belief that environment and engagement are crucially important for people with dementia. Still, it was striking to see such profound improvement, so quickly, with simple interventions. It encouraged our team to believe that change was achievable. We started to understand, in practical terms, that so many of the behaviours causing problems in health and aged care services are a function of people being placed in restrictive environments and encountering staff responses that exacerbate problems.

❖❖❖

Following the Oakden Report, the issue of having CCTV installed in aged care environments intensified as a topic of public debate. There had already been a highly publicised incident in another Adelaide residential aged care facility. Noleen Hausler had been so worried about the care of her father, who had dementia, that she secretly installed a camera in his room, only to film a horrendous assault by a care worker when he was meant to be assisting Noleen's father during a meal. The footage of the incident – which was distressing to watch – was shown on prime-time news broadcasts and re-emerged after the Oakden Report, and during the Royal Commission into Aged Care Quality and Safety, which coincided with the trial – and conviction – of the care worker involved.[6] It all served to heighten the anxiety felt by families and staff across the sector.

At Northgate House, the organisation had already installed CCTV into all the common areas prior to us moving in. There were concerns raised by staff regarding the presence of these cameras and, given the punitive tone of the early post-Oakden period, this was understandable. Following an industrial process, an approach to the use of CCTV was agreed. Staff quickly got used to it being in place, and business continued with the cameras unnoticed. There are more innovative technologies that can support safety in aged care settings with less compromise of privacy, however we found the CCTV to be a useful tool in understanding several early incidents as we continued our process of change. It helped clarify situations where there was a question over how staff members were managing challenges in practice. It provided data that facilitated much more accurate debriefing, reflection and learning.

One such incident occurred about six months after we had moved into Northgate House. We were making progress, but still had a long way to go. Vera, our resident from Oakden with severe schizoaffective disorder, presented with one of her recurrent episodes where she became very depressed, with dark, persecutory beliefs of being in personal danger. During these episodes, she would become highly agitated, yell at other residents and staff and, in her efforts to ensure her own safety, sometimes behave aggressively. Vera did not intend to hurt anyone and, if she did, she would later tearfully apologise. But after many years of institutional living, she did not mind causing damage to property. Vera worked out how to angle a chair or table to crack through the strong glass panels in the expanse of windows in the main living area. She did this several times before we developed a sustainable plan to reduce risk by giving Vera enough space to calm herself down.

One evening, at the start of this learning process, Vera became agitated. She started voicing delusional ideas about other residents and some of the staff. Without moving from a lounge chair in the main living area, she made stammered threats about 'getting' another resident she perceived as a threat who, by that time, was asleep in bed. The staff became alarmed and started a process of escalation, which led to the police and an ambulance being called – all while Vera remained in her seat in the lounge.

A steep and strenuous climb

The CCTV showed how the situation snowballed, driven by staff anxiety without any real action from Vera. After several hours, the ambulance and police officers arrived to transport Vera to the hospital for an acute assessment. One of the ambulance officers spoke with Vera, who was still just sitting in her chair, displaying no physically aggressive behaviour. But the cascade had already commenced. The ambulance officer looked around to see who was in charge and what to do next. No one took the lead. Nobody had the confidence to call a stop and re-evaluate.

Two breathtakingly tall police officers stepped out from behind her chair, suddenly coming into Vera's line of sight. They took hold of an arm each and applied handcuffs, joining Vera's wrists together. At that point, Vera finally reacted. She started kicking, squirming and trying to bite. In fairness, she was defending herself.

Vera soon gave in and stood up; her hands cuffed in front of her. She shuffled over to the waiting barouche. She was helped on by the ambulance officers, who then 'netted' her, applying firm elastic over her body to immobilise her. Familiar with the indignity afforded her in a health system that failed to understand her, or hold the anxiety she provoked, Vera acquiesced. She went to the hospital, was detained under the Mental Health Act, and the following day, after the order was revoked, returned to Northgate House to sit once again on her preferred lounge chair.

We used the CCTV footage to debrief as a team. The ambulance service joined us. We were all shocked and disappointed at how we had functioned as services; at how quick our teams had been to escalate responses, and how we lacked the confidence to slow down, watch and wait. It was bizarre and unjust that a seventy-something-year-old woman with limited physical ability had triggered such a reactive and restrictive response from health providers. We recognised how easy it was to see Vera as an awkward 'other', to miss her story and overlook her humanity. How often does this happen at interpersonal junction points in our lives, especially those that confront us with difference and discomfort?

We used the incident as a turning point, firstly in care planning for Vera, and secondly in the way we delivered care as a whole team. The ambos did the same. Vera's mental state continued to fluctuate over the remainder of her life, but she was *never* handcuffed, netted or transferred to the hospital again.

Our fledgling service gradually found its way. Instead of complaints, we started to receive compliments and thanks from family members. There was a tangible improvement in the care delivered and received every day. Our team was still fractured and shaken but we had, finally, begun the steep and strenuous climb out of Oakden.

11

Politicians and persuasion

On my way up the steep learning curve through crisis and scandal, I was struck by the presence of distinct, yet interacting, narratives. One of these was the political drama that unfolded alongside the day-to-day realities of the people who lived and worked in the service. Politics is a difficult business. It's populated with talented, well-intentioned people who aspire to lead positive change. At the same time, it carries the risk of hubris, of being unable to accept and acknowledge failure, and having to manage the pressures of public perception through the never-ending work of spin. As I tried to make sense of my observations of this political universe, someone sagely said to me, 'That's just politicians doing what politicians do.'

Yet there are important lessons here too, embedded in stories. To explore these, it's necessary to backtrack in time to pick up a different view, starting once again in those early weeks after I arrived at Oakden and slipped over on the gleaming vinyl floor.

❖❖❖

My phone rang. It was a number I didn't recognise. 'Hello,' I answered. A friendly, confident voice greeted me.

'Hi Duncan, it's Alex.'

Alex spoke like a long-lost friend, as if I knew exactly who she was. I had no idea.

'You know …' she went on, clearly sensing my confusion, '… the advisor, from the minister's team. We met the other day.'

'Oh yes,' I replied, desperately trying to locate her face in my overwhelmed memory.

Just days before, the premier, the Honourable Jay Weatherill, MP, had visited Oakden. I was in the office when Jackie Hanson walked in.

'We're not meant to know this,' she said, 'but the premier's coming, unannounced.'

'Oh my!' I gasped. 'When?'

'Now,' came the answer. 'He's about ten minutes away.'

We were busy. It felt like we were interrupted every five minutes to respond to another demand. Again, there was the irony that an institution that had been invisible and neglected for more than fifteen years was now inundated by dignitaries wanting to witness scenes they might have taken an interest in a thousand times before. Of course, it was wholly appropriate for the premier to come, and I was glad of the opportunity to talk about what we needed.

A cavalcade of security, advisors and staff surrounded the premier. Minister for Mental Health, Leesa Vlahos, walked beside him, explaining bits and pieces of detail as they went. Apart from the premier and the minister, I was not sure who I met that day. The premier was gracious, asserting his commitment that what had occurred at Oakden would be put right, no matter what the cost.

I am not sure that he fully comprehended the complex needs of the population at Oakden, and it may have been unreasonable to expect this of him. Still, he appeared to listen and engage, probing with questions.

Days later, when the advisor rang me, I was unprepared. Multiple narratives were evolving. An election would be held in less than a year and, for the government, there was much at stake. A scandal was breaking – in which I was a player and therefore fair game for such conversations.

I have never been able to discipline myself long enough to hold a poker face, much preferring to wear my heart on my sleeve. I would be poorly suited to politics because of this. I spoke far too candidly to the advisor about my impressions after my first weeks at the epicentre of the crisis.

I had been perturbed by the degree of reactivity, involving punitive responses and knee-jerk decisions that lacked engagement with the people who would be affected by them. I had been bothered by the lack of consideration for sustainability beyond the immediate public crisis. I was too open with the information I had acquired, with no awareness of how a seasoned political player might use it. I blithely recounted everything from my observations to the gossip I had heard about people making backroom deals. It was like being caught up in a daytime TV soap opera. Concurrently, there were real lives and stories that needed to be fully understood and managed with timely and sustainable dignity and care.

❖❖❖

In my first week in the job, I had found myself compelled to respond to this drama of extreme reactivity. The media had reported another incident of alleged misconduct by a staff member. While I will never know the premier's exact words, by the time I was brought up to speed, he had reportedly issued a directive that no one was safe in Oakden, and we were to move everyone out of there by the following day.

The Chief Executive had already pushed back against the idea. There was no way it could be done, and nor was it necessary – or safe. Nonetheless, there was an expectation that consideration should be given to identifying alternative environments that could rapidly facilitate a mass decanting of residents from Oakden. I suspect the unconscious drive was to close the facility and run away from all it represented as quickly as possible.

The other part of the directive, equally unrealistic, was that none of the staff should be included in the transfer to a new site. It was a misreading of the situation to suggest that all staff were abusive. There were issues of industrial legislation and principles of natural justice that needed to be observed. It would have been an untenable solution to simply move all the residents to a hospital, and equally ridiculous to assume that there would be purpose-ready new staff waiting to take over what was probably the least appealing job in the country at the time.

Despite my protestations that this was lunacy, I was bundled into a government car with the Executive Director of Infrastructure, and Chief Psychiatrist Aaron Groves. We drove to several disused, decommissioned and antiquated Department of Health-owned sites, scoping for viable alternative campuses. One of the sites was on an upper floor of a building used since the 1960s for people with disabilities – previously called the 'Home for Incurables'. It was coming to the end of its days for that purpose, and the asbestos-riddled space we reviewed was entirely unsuitable for providing care for people with dementia.

We clambered through neglected gardens at another site to review cottage-style accommodation, previously used for people with disabilities but now having lain unused for a decade. The buildings were broken down and filthy. As we entered one cottage there was a scurry of activity as rats and cockroaches dived for cover. It dawned on me that I was caught up in the most ridiculous farce.

My phone rang. It was the Chief Executive.

'It can't be done,' I assured her. 'This has been a waste of time, and if we continue in this direction, we'll only do more harm to the people at Oakden.'

'Good,' said the CE. 'That's what I need to hear.'

'What's more,' I continued, gaining confidence, 'I can't do this job if they're going to be making decisions like this.'

'Well, hold steady,' she said. 'Hopefully there won't be any need for that. I just need to be able to say that we've had the clinical advice, and a move is not possible – or safe.'

It was only one day of my life, traipsing around the city on a goose chase. The CE pushed back; the premier took a breath and gave us a reprieve. A more reasonable decision was taken to progress with the renovation at Northgate. This was underway when I took the call from the advisor and over-disclosed all that was crashing through my mind. It was not the last call: we had several subsequent conversations focused on managing the evolving narrative, and in this I learnt an important lesson about knowing and doing my own business.

❖❖❖

There were multiple families of Oakden residents, past and present, speaking with the media. These families had experienced trauma and grief. Sometimes their distress spilled out in interviews, with allegations against nurses, doctors, the health system and the government. Their outrage threatened to become overwhelming, derailing the delicately managed drama.

To soothe the storm of emotions, and reflecting genuine regret that the situation had occurred, promises and assurances were offered to these families by politicians and echoed by executives. Families frequently referred to the premier's reassurances that there would be no personal or financial disadvantage.

'Money is no problem,' he was cited as saying. 'We will make this right.'

The problem was that there was no concurrent counting of the cost – thinking about what was practically possible, or how recovery would be sustained. Promises are taken seriously by the people to whom they are made. But in all aspects of government and public health, money is always a problem, and it sets up false hope to suggest otherwise. What was needed was a clear plan, built on evidence, with well-developed strategy, accurately costed up and commissioned – and then honestly articulated. By contrast, the politics of the situation tumbled along in a reactionary manner, managing crisis after crisis, and responding to feedback from media-active families.

I found myself in a predicament. I was trying to make appropriate clinical decisions around each person's care, identifying what they needed and titrating this against available resources. Many of the residents' needs had changed since their admission to Oakden, due to the natural progression of dementia. It was reasonable to support their transition to mainstream aged care homes – the work being undertaken with skill and efficiency by Jacqui and Claire.

We were commissioning only sixteen places of care in the Northgate renovation, while closing sixty-four places at Oakden. This was, in itself, an illustration of how governments and executives make reactive decisions without fully thinking through the implications. We could not possibly accommodate everyone – and yet families had reasonable expectations based on assurances they had been given. To disappoint media-active families had the potential to be politically compromising.

One such family had been through the most challenging of experiences, involving an allegation of undue force against their mother, Mrs Donaldson, by a staff member. They were angry, and rightly so. But in their heartache, they struggled to differentiate between the wrongs at Oakden and their beloved mother's contemporary needs. Mrs Donaldson had entered Oakden because she had dementia, complicated by aggressive behaviour. On at least one occasion, possibly more, her care had been horribly mismanaged, leading to direct and inexcusable trauma. But by the time I took over her care, the behavioural symptoms that had resulted in her admission to Oakden were long gone. She could no longer talk or walk and was completely dependent on others. She no longer required care in a specialist service; her care needs could now be met in a quality aged care home. Mrs Donaldson was approaching the end of her life, and there was more risk of another person with dementia causing her harm by staying where she was.

But her family members were anxious about what might happen in a mainstream facility because of their previous experiences in aged care (when her clinical presentation had been much more complex and challenging). They felt that the whole health and aged care system had let them down, and that was fair enough. The consequence was that they held unrealistic expectations, driven by hurt and anxiety, which threatened to spill out in a hard-to-contain media story.

Enter stage left: Alex, the advisor, capable of managing almost any sensitive storyline.

I had worked hard with Mrs Donaldson's family, supporting them through grieving, letting go of their anger, and accepting a transition. It was a difficult time for them, and they remained brittle. I had no idea that in parallel with this, the family were also having separate conversations with the advisor, and that alternative undertakings were being made.

I received another call from the advisor. 'Mrs Donaldson's family are so worried – they've been through so much,' she said. 'Is there any way you can find a way to accommodate their mother at Northgate House? It would be so much better.'

The conversation went back and forth. I was weighing up options on the fly – trying to work out who needed access to the service and who could safely and reasonably be offered an alternative pathway. Being eager to please, I gave in to the advisor and agreed that we would offer Mrs Donaldson a place at Northgate House – a decision that would come back to bite me.

As the opening of Northgate House grew closer, the limitations on capacity became painfully evident. I quickly realised that I had made a mistake. More people had been promised places of care than we had available. Taking with me a large slice of humble pie, I went back to Mrs Donaldson's family, apologetic but needing to revisit the issue of transitioning to a place in a mainstream aged care home. They were extremely reluctant to accept this and cited the advisor's promises. It got messy. There were more negotiations, more conversations back and forth with the advisor. The family eventually, but reluctantly, accepted the mainstream aged care place offered to them. Mrs Donaldson transitioned successfully, but quickly progressed to the end of her life.

Then, just when it looked like the situation had been resolved, one of Mrs Donaldson's family members suddenly appeared on a current affairs TV program, a shadowy, de-identifed image, tearfully describing their mother's trauma at Oakden. They told how the 'head psychiatrist' had made promises that were not kept. It was mortifying. I felt humiliated. I had no right of reply. I wanted to explain that I had made an error in judgement, giving in to pressure to help manage the political fallout but failing the person at the centre of care by neglecting to speak honestly. We weathered this storm as a service, and I learnt that quality clinical decision-making needs to be kept separate from politics.

❖❖❖

Fast-forward several months and the investigation by Bruce Lander, QC, the Independent Commissioner Against Corruption (ICAC), regarding who was responsible for Oakden, was underway. The Commissioner's role was to protect the integrity of public administration, and this was his most sensational case.

There was public controversy over whether the Commissioner should hold open public hearings, or whether they should remain closed. Public hearings would have been potentially embarrassing and therefore disadvantageous to the government. The premier was clear that the review would be conducted behind closed doors. No Cabinet documents were to be released to the investigation.[1] The opposition's view differed: they called for open hearings.[2] There was a possibility that the hearings would cause significant stress to specific individuals, and this needed consideration. But if we take the politics of pending elections out of the picture, and consider values of honesty and integrity, there was a robust argument for bringing everything into the light and allowing the public to come in. I wonder, if the positions of government and opposition had been reversed, whether both sides would have changed their perspectives?

The ICAC Report was released in mid-February 2018, just weeks before the state election. Many people in the community may have wondered if the proximity of the report's release to the state election was coincidental, or some kind of statement on the Commissioner's part. There was no mistaking the Commissioner's intent in his choice of title: *Oakden: A Shameful Chapter in South Australia's History*.[3]

The report itself was controversial. It took a mostly punitive stance – which makes sense in many ways – but in my view did not aim its findings at a sufficiently senior level. When five people local to the service at Oakden were found guilty of maladministration, including my predecessor, but no executive or politician was directly called to account, it was a bitter pill for staff working at the coalface. They knew there had been serial neglect from multiple executives and politicians who had failed to take an interest in the vulnerable people at Oakden and the service tasked with accommodating them.

To his credit, the Commissioner acknowledged that his findings 'did not tell the entire story'. He expressed 'astonishment' that 'senior people, including ministers and chief executives, who were responsible by virtue of their office for the delivery of care and services to the consumers at the Oakden facility, should have known what was going on but did not'.[4]

In his public statement responding to the ICAC Report, the premier asserted that the government accepted full responsibility for what had happened at Oakden.[5] The key points, picked up and disseminated by the media, from the premier's press conference in February 2018, appeared to be carefully crafted:

> *It was shameful. What happened at Oakden must never be repeated. These patients were vulnerable South Australians. The abuse that they suffered at the hands of the workers that were meant to care for them was abhorrent. The inability of the agency to detect and prevent that abuse is unacceptable.*
>
> *To anyone who suffered abuse at the hands of the workers at Oakden, I am deeply sorry ...*
>
> *They all deserved better from the workers at this government agency and those who were meant to supervise them.*
>
> *My government's policy has always been zero tolerance for elder abuse.*
>
> *The Commissioner finds that no Minister was aware of the nature and extent of the abuse at Oakden. He also finds that, had they been aware, they would have taken steps to remedy it.*
>
> *But they should have been told.*[6]

Granted, there was an apology – but what was *heard* by the public, and particularly by the staff who remained at the frontline, trying to undertake the work of reform, was that it was aberrant care staff who were to blame, or the quality agency for not picking up the problems. What was *not heard* was transparent ownership of the government's lack of interest and inactivity – of the barriers to them *being told*. I noted the irony, given my previous trips to the ministers' offices with the College of Psychiatrists. By implication, how could the premier and his government be accountable for the actions of some terrible nurses and their incompetent managers in an isolated backwater?

The opposition must have been dancing in their campaign office.

'If anybody needs any proof whatsoever that this is the worst government in the State's history,' declared opposition leader Steven Marshall after the report's release, 'they can read about it today.'

To avoid confusion, he summarised the findings: 'Labor has failed our most vulnerable citizens – they deserve to be sacked ... every South Australian should be outraged.'[7]

Another person whose fate was sealed by the ICAC Report was the former Minister for Mental Health, Leesa Vlahos. Things had gone from bad to worse for her over many months. She stepped down as minister but remained at the top of the Labor ticket for the South Australian legislative council. There was much speculation in the weeks preceding the ICAC Report's release around her being a liability for the government. The polls indicated a pending defeat at the forthcoming election. We can only imagine the conversations that were held behind closed doors. Two weeks before the report's release, Leesa Vlahos resigned from politics, announcing her withdrawal from the election.

The evidence in the ICAC Report suggested that Vlahos had not helped her cause, and the Commissioner was merciless in assessing her. Vlahos had publicly claimed that she commissioned the Oakden Report – the Commissioner found that she did not and that this was the work of Jackie Hanson. Lander exposed Vlahos as a prevaricator.

'She did not lead in addressing the crisis,' he judged. 'She followed.'

He described her as a 'very poor witness' who was 'sullen and surly', 'belligerent and aggressive', 'deliberately untruthful', and 'inherently inconsistent'. She was infamously reported to have shouted at the Commissioner and blamed others.[8]

With the ICAC Report released and Leesa Vlahos' political career concluded, I was summoned to a meeting with the premier, the recently appointed Minister for Health and Mental Health, Peter Malinauskas, and their teams, and the publicly active Oakden families – a meeting convened by the premier to respond to the ICAC Report. There was minimal briefing provided. I turned up at the premier's office suited up and, by that stage, jaded by the process.

As I waited in a corridor, the premier and his team were in a briefing room, watching the early news reports – no doubt gauging the likely temperature of media-cultivated public opinion. After the news had finished, they emerged from the briefing room, and I was shown into a large meeting room with a table around which Cabinet would normally sit. I sat next to the premier and the minister.

The families were ushered in and filled the remaining seats. Among them was the family member of Mrs Donaldson, the Oakden resident who had transitioned to a residential aged care facility rather than Northgate House. The government staffers stood around the room. Alex, the advisor, with whom I'd had many phone conversations regarding Mrs Donaldson, stood a little behind me.

There was tension in the meeting room. The view held by many of the family members was that not enough had been done to bring offending staff to justice. For these people, because of what they had suffered personally, the identification of guilty individuals – particularly direct care staff – seemed to take precedence over remediation of system failures. Families called for prosecutions against staff, sackings, and assurance that they would never work again.

The premier assured the families that problem staff would be dealt with. He did not say how.

What was happening by then, was that nearly thirty staff had been stepped down from work at Oakden, and there were ongoing legal and registration processes progressing around many of these. Some staff had chosen to leave. Other staff who had worked at Oakden continued in the new service – most of whom were caring, good-quality staff who raised no cause for concern. By this time, we had also recruited many new staff. There was inadequate time and space to explain all this – especially when the predominating mood felt more like baying for blood.

Attention in the meeting shifted to perceived failures in the government's handling of the scandal. The families were dissatisfied. They alleged that Leesa Vlahos had falsely reassured them. Damned by her portrayal in the ICAC Report, she emerged as a culpable figure who had failed to manage the crisis. It seemed as if the premier seized the opportunity to extricate himself and direct blame as far as possible from the remainder of the government.

'That's why she's no longer a member of my government,' I recall him declaring.

At the premier's press conference earlier the same day, it had been a similar picture. When confronted with his previous defence of the minister, he appeared flummoxed and then described her behaviour as 'unacceptable'.

'She's no longer a candidate for the Labor Party,' he confirmed.[9]

You could almost hear the bus wheels crunching her bones as he chucked her under it. Politics is a harsh world, particularly for women. Months earlier, the premier had stood behind the minister in her troubles. Now she was a liability, and it appeared there was no mercy.

Back in the meeting with the families, the focus shifted toward the process of positive change that had begun. The premier asked me to talk about efforts in closing Oakden and opening Northgate House. It went well enough, until Mrs Donaldson's family member suddenly launched into a furious tirade.

'You *lied* to me, Duncan. You lied!'

I was taken aback.

The tirade continued: 'You told me my mother had a place at Northgate, and then you made us take some place at a facility, where they just let her sit in a chair and do nothing.'

The family member was red-faced and shedding angry tears by the end of this.

I tried to explain the context of what had happened, remaining outwardly gracious and calm. But I did not feel calm on the inside. In a momentary flash of dissociative illusion, I imagined myself turning to point at the advisor, saying, 'Wait a minute … I tried to do the right thing, but I made a mistake. See that person back there? They got me to agree to your request when I knew it was impossible from the beginning!'

I desperately wanted to set the record straight – as inappropriate as that would have been. It was just as well that it was easier to imagine than to do. The truth is, Alex the advisor had been doing her job, with the best of intentions, just as I had. If only we had both slowed things down earlier.

Another family member, who had actively engaged with the post-Oakden reform process came to my rescue. I was profoundly grateful for a supportive voice. 'Don't go after Duncan,' he said, 'he's one of the good guys. He's working hard to fix the problem, so don't shoot *him*.'

❖❖❖

It seemed to me that several different narratives were sitting around the table that afternoon, competing for dominance. From where I sat, the ascendent political narrative appeared characterised by the ascription of blame – to service staff, managers, accreditors, anyone – to mitigate the government's accountability. I found that the way the former minister so wholly and rapidly became an outsider – an 'other' – was disturbing. I felt as though the noble task of leading and governing was obscured by the need to manage public perception and voter intention. This insight into the machinations of spin, deployed to persuade people that the government was not only *not* responsible for what had happened but was, in fact, *responsibly responsive* (rather than acknowledge that this failure had sat under its nose for more than a decade), was deeply disheartening. I did not see this as an issue of party politics but rather as a function of the political world itself, the pressures of which drive politicians towards such ways of behaving as a means of survival. They are at the mercy of how they are portrayed and perceived as they are confronted with complex problems. This does not support the simplicity of a transparent apology.

But as I sat at that table on that particular day, the influence of persuasion was such that I felt it impossible to voice objection to this rendition of the story. With the charismatic personalities and machinery of government looming all around me, and a belief that I needed their support to achieve the reform outcomes I was working toward, I struggled with feelings of intimidation and powerlessness. I could sense the pressure to comply and the expectation to spruik the party line; I was aware of the professional risk if I were to challenge the preferred narrative. While I earnestly hoped that everyone had learnt the real lessons that Oakden had to teach, I felt the main issue on the table was managing the fallout. And in my disquiet were sown the seeds of cynicism and burnout.

In further parallel to these tough lessons about the politics of a public scandal, I found another nexus of learning – and personal unease – in my interactions with the media, with whom the government and its spin doctors were compelled to engage in an intricate two-step. Here I witnessed the construction and dissemination of a public narrative that often deviated from a balanced telling of the real stories of what happened at Oakden.

12

Media and messaging

I have seldom struggled with words. There was one painfully awkward moment in a Year 10 interhouse debate where my mind went strangely blank. I said my first and only public-speaking swearword and everyone waited awkwardly for my three-minute train wreck to be over. Oh, Lord! The memory! Other than that, I have typically been able to find appropriate words in most situations.

Words tell stories, communicate perspectives, and create perceived realities. When we wrote the Oakden Report, we did not anticipate the creation of narrative worlds – in personal, political, and public domains – that emerged in the aftermath of the report's release. Prominent among these was a public narrative generated by voracious journalists and producers, who had caught the scent of a drama and circled it relentlessly.

Before 2017, I had never participated in a press conference – although neither had I been caught up in the middle of a national scandal. The local Bathurst newspaper, the *Western Advocate*, interviewed me a couple of times as a school student – a highlight of my life at the time. Many years later, when I found myself trundled out in front of cameras, microphones and reporters, I needed to rely on my ability to string words together instinctively. I did not undertake any media training until the crisis was mostly over – by which time the media was less interested in asking me questions.

To start with, I was unaware that I was now a cast member, with a particular role, in a piece of improvisational theatre played out between politicians and their advisors, and the unremitting media. In this drama, I was the trusted clinician – apolitical, with an honest face and sincere manner – whose role was to reassure the public that the failings of Oakden would never happen again. I inhabited the role with complete conviction.

There were other players in the drama. There was Leesa Vlahos, the minister, on the back foot from the start and ultimately to play the pariah; the premier and the government, clinging to long-held power; the opposition, sensing that this could be the issue to drive home a long-denied election victory; and there was a group of families who became the faces of Oakden and represented a narrative of abuse and harm.

It appeared that our roles were assigned. The story played out in the public domain, conveyed by reporters and news producers; a created product that captured neither nuances nor the whole truth. Instead, it became a dichotomous tale, with villains and victims, where the villains were the frontline clinical staff or selected scapegoats, such as the minister.

The Mid Staffordshire Report in the UK triggered an aspiration for the NHS to shift from a 'blame culture to a learning culture'.[1] It is hard to achieve a learning culture while the preeminent narrative is an endless hunt for blame.

'The burning question about the Oakden nursing home scandal,' declared one of the news by-lines, 'is who is ultimately responsible – and who should, quite rightly, lose their jobs?'[2]

Whilst a retrospective analysis of accountability had its place, a dialogue about how we could carve out a secure future through positive service reform would have been more meaningful.

This tension between learning and blame resulted in a paradox. On the one hand, the media was an essential player in the drama, generating enough attention to ensure that Oakden remained on the public and political agendas. I will remain forever grateful for the media influence that made the health and dignity of older people a public concern. The story was launched by ABC reporters Nicola Gage and Angelique Donnellan, who had forged a trusting relationship with Barb Spriggs. They presented a candid but well-measured account of the saga, and later shared a human rights journalism award nomination in 2017 and won a public service journalism award in 2018 for their work on the story.[3]

On the other hand, the media, in general, struggled to tell the whole truth of the story. Being on the inside, I often identified errors and misquotes in the reporting of details. This bothered me. Further, it seemed that the quest for theatre and sensation influenced the tone of the narrative. Adjectives such as 'infamous' and 'shocking' predominated and affected how the story was understood.

Prior to the closure of Oakden, the media confronted staff as they turned up to work in the morning. Reporters attempted to break into the facility after hours. On one occasion, a man delivered a pizza to the door at 3 am. No one had ordered pizza. It turned out he was a journalist trying to get inside with his camera. Another time, a well-meaning family member smuggled a reporter in during a visit. The reporter scouted around, taking pictures of residents, before being identified and asked to leave. This behaviour was clearly outside of journalistic ethics.

It was a siege that seemed to last for an eternity. Over the weeks, and then months, the headlines continued: 'Widow recalls husband's horror death';[4] 'Our day of shame';[5] 'One of Australia's greatest disgraces'.[6]

Arguably all true. Nonetheless, from where I sat, it seemed all the more of an uphill struggle to articulate a voice of reform in the face of an incessant and provocative narrative of shame and failure. It made it more challenging to express the truth of what had happened on a systems level. Perceived solutions to problems were over-simplified. It was never going to be as straightforward or unsophisticated as replacing all the nursing staff. There was more to it than that.

AN EVERYONE STORY

❖❖❖

My first press conference was on a Sunday morning in June 2017, shortly before we opened Northgate House, facilitating the closure of the wards at Oakden. The rapid-fire refurbishment was complete. With the first transition of residents just days away, a press conference had been organised for the minister and me to talk to the media, and to provide reporters and families of Oakden residents with a tour of the new facility.

The morning of the press conference, I was terrified. I put on my tie and jacket and arrived on site early. The manager of the refurbishment was putting last-minute touches to the unit. Despite being overcast, the site appeared warm, light, and comfortable – a significant improvement to Oakden.

CEO Jackie Hanson and executives from the local health network arrived, followed by the minister, Leesa Vlahos, and her team, including her policy and media advisors. I put on a 'sure-I'm-fine' face, but I remained nervous. I was, after all, hanging out with the minister and the network executives, getting ready to be on TV – I had slipped into an alternate reality.

All the major television networks turned up. They were corralled outside before being ushered into the unit at the designated time. They set up in a semicircle in the lounge area. For the first time, I had the surreal experience of being instructed to keep looking straight ahead at a camera. At the same time, the reporters, flanking each side of us, pushed microphones towards us and peppered us with questions, initially aimed at the minister and then at me. I kept getting redirected because I was unable to resist the temptation to turn toward the journalist who had asked a question and talk to them as another human being.

There was so much going on inside my head. Despite the awkwardness, I tried to be honest, no matter what they asked. At the same time, I tried to remain positive, earnestly hoping that we were at the start of a process that would continue unabated until the work of reform was fully implemented.

Media and messaging

The minister had a hard time. The tone of questions directed at her was, at best, assertive, at worst, accusatory. It was deeply uncomfortable. Just like my painful Year 10 debating debacle, I think everyone watching hoped for it to be over soon. I initially fared better. My script was more straightforward: we needed to provide quality care to people with complex needs, and we were getting on with the job.

But then I was asked the questions that would subsequently arise at every opportunity. How many incidents of staff abusing residents had occurred? How many staff had been reported to the police? How many staff had been stood down? How many staff from Oakden would be working at Northgate? These questions became the focus of the media's reporting.

I knew that workplace culture was a primary issue that profoundly influenced the behaviour of staff and the delivery of care. Still, to tar all Oakden staff with one brush was a misrepresentation and missed the point of the reform process. I did my best to answer these questions with patience and candour, but over the months, they became increasingly frustrating.

❖ ❖ ❖

'Going viral' is a phenomenon in the modern world. In an era of social media, we all know that a simple, well-phrased meme or captivating image can have an expansive impact. As the minister encountered intensifying scrutiny, an unfortunate photograph of her vigorously flinging a large plastic fish – a publicity stunt at the South Australian Tunarama Festival – took on a life of its own. Fortuitous for the media, the phrase 'the fish rots from the head', quoted in the Oakden Report about the finding of a failure of governance, provided the perfect caption to the image, which appeared in papers and online.[7] Leesa Vlahos' life was becoming increasingly difficult.

The minister was hammered about what she knew and when. Accounts of what might otherwise have been justifiable political jaunts overseas or to cultural events, such as the celebration of the fishing industry, were portrayed by the media as insensitive and irresponsible blunders. The image of her hurling the fish played perfectly into the archetype of Nero fiddling while Rome turned to cinders. It was a story generated in the public domain by media story-makers, and it became destructive beyond the degree of recrimination deserved by the minister. I'm not suggesting that she made no errors, but as a study in bad timing, she carried the can for a whole series of ministers and executives, any of whom might have acted but did not. If we are honest, that was not fair – but it was how the story was told.

❖❖❖

Some months later, the minister resigned. She moved to the backbench, on her way out of politics altogether. She was replaced as Minister for Mental Health by the young, charismatic, good-looking and talented Peter Malinauskas ('Pete'), who also picked up the health portfolio – I had no doubt that he was future premier material. Malinauskas had acumen and assurance that had eluded his predecessor. On his first visit to Northgate House, surrounded by his team of equally youthful, good-looking and go-getting male staffers, he was highly personable and asked perceptive questions.

'Minister,' I greeted him as he arrived.

'Doctor,' he responded with feigned gravity, and then laughed.

I showed him around the home. As we walked through the gardens of the women's house, one of the residents – Molly, a sixty-something-year-old woman with frontotemporal dementia that resulted in disinhibition, overeating and being generally larger than life – saw the visiting group of handsome young men. She made a beeline for them, hitching her dress at her hips and calling out, 'Well hello, boys!'

The minister and his team were suitably gracious, almost a touch playful back. Molly was delighted. She commented on their youthful good looks and, just to be clear, turned to me and said, 'But not you ...'

Everyone laughed – and I accepted being put in my place.

A short while after Malinauskas became minister, an incident garnered media attention. An old-school mental health nurse had returned to work after extended leave, having been away since before the Oakden review. The nurse arrived on a night shift during the highly disruptive period of change that surrounded the establishment of Northgate House.

Vera, our resident with severe schizoaffective disorder, was quite unwell at the time and was expressing jumbled ideas about being under attack from all sorts of people, including staff. She yelled abusively at some of the staff, including the newly returned mental health nurse.

Some staff were now recognising that Vera did much better when given space and quiet, rather than having people get in her way as they tried to talk her down. By leaving her to sit quietly, uninterrupted, potential risks of her hurting someone else could be reduced by supporting other residents to give her a wide berth. A crisis management plan was developing around the idea that, with the right environment and support, Vera could de-escalate herself.

Unfortunately, on this occasion, there was no wide berth or space given to Vera. I was on call. At about midnight, I received a phone call from the mental health nurse, letting me know that approximately two hours earlier, staff had managed Vera's reported high-risk, aggressive behaviour by physically restraining her and administering an intramuscular injection. Vera was a woman in her seventies, heavy-set and slowed with a shuffling gait. The story did not make sense. Troubled by this, I asked multiple questions, trying to find out what had happened and why. The following day, I began an investigation into the incident, including a review of the CCTV footage.

The footage was telling. Rather than retreating and providing space, the mental health nurse had assumed a dominant posture, standing over Vera, pointing at her, giving her instructions, and expecting compliance. The nurse signalled for other, less experienced nurses to take positions at four corners around Vera. They placed a chair in front of Vera as a barrier, edging this toward her. Unquestionably, she felt intimidated. She pushed the chair back toward the nurse, albeit with limited force. There was a significant disparity between the evidence available on CCTV and the dramatic description of running amok in the incident report.

Just as she had experienced when being frog-marched to the bathroom at Oakden, Vera was held firmly by the nurses. The group tramped her around to her room, where she disappeared from the CCTV record. The mental health nurse followed the nurses into the room with a prepared syringe of medication drawn up in his pocket. It appeared the decision to administer the intramuscular injection had been made sometime earlier. The statements of the other nurses indicated that Vera was held on the bed and given the injection. She was then left in her room and was finally able to calm down.

The investigation determined that the mental health nurse had not technically done anything incorrect. It was true that Vera had been unwell at the time. She had made confronting verbal statements to staff. She had pushed the chair back toward the nurse. The intramuscular medication had been charted on her 'as required' medication chart, reflecting the hangover of previous ways of managing her care. This was ceased quickly after the incident to prevent a repetition.

But these factors do not make what happened okay. The problem was one of culture and practice. The incident reflected an antiquated, institutional, and clinically punitive approach to care in which the 'patient' was regarded as the problem: the phenomenon of 'othering'.

Addressing this was the real work that was needed. It meant finding the space to engage with the workforce, deal with things constructively, articulate a better way to work, build trust and change culture. It was even more challenging to manage these issues against the backdrop of sensational media reporting, where an incident such as this served to reinforce public assumptions about the staff.

As was routine practice in the immediate post-Oakden era, the incident resulted in a police report including questions about whether any aspect of the incident should be construed as an assault. The legal advice was that it should not. Randomly, a journalist rang the police asking about other matters and, for whatever reason, the police officer mentioned that there was a new investigation into an incident at Northgate House involving a former Oakden staff member. This was a red rag to a bull, and within hours there was a flurry of media reports on the latest incident related to Oakden.

An inner voice prompted me to wear a suit and tie to work the following day, not my usual practice. Just as well. At about midday, I received a call from the minister's office. My presence was requested for a meeting about the incident. The minister, I was informed, would be meeting the media for a press conference later that day.

The office was an expansive room on the ninth floor of the Department of Health building, with two window-filled walls providing panoramic views across to the Adelaide Hills. The mood was intense and had the tone of a war-room briefing.

I felt like a fish scooped out of a pond and plonked onto a rock. My first task was to clarify what had occurred during the incident. I duly obliged, but – quite understandably – the minister and his team appeared less focused on understanding the actual events and were more concerned about the potential onslaught from the reporters who, as we talked, were already gathering in the street below.

There was discussion about what should and should not be disclosed. At one point, I innocently suggested that perhaps we should just tell the truth. The minister had more extensive experience of such matters and pointed out that the truth was not the primary interest of the press, who were stamping their feet on the pavement, eager for a story replete with as much scandal as possible.

The minister was right. As we faced them outside, it was evident that the reporters wanted drama. After months of conflict, I was tired, and my resilience was reduced. Unconsciously, I drifted into a surreal and dissociated glaze. It was as if I had stepped out of my body and was surveying the scene from a little way off. Everything moved more slowly, and I found myself listening to the minister and the reporters as if I were underwater. I suddenly realised that, at any moment, I would be asked a question. Like pushing upward through the water to break the surface, I forced myself to reconnect with the moment. Within seconds, a reporter turned to me to ask the same questions as always: 'Did the staff member involved work at Oakden?' 'How many staff at Northgate House worked at Oakden?' 'How can you be sure this will not happen again?'

It seemed impossible to describe events in a way that accurately represented what had occurred – what the person at the centre of the incident had experienced, or the nurses who found themselves caught up in it. There was no opportunity to clarify what was meant by restrictive practices – that these are sometimes used, regrettably, but should be actively avoided. It did not mean that a staff member had hit a patient, which was the assumption made at the press conference. There was no platform for a nuanced explanation that acknowledged systematic disinvestment, demoralised culture, and the undermining of human dignity over the years. None of these make for a snappy sound bite or captivating TV.

I started to resent the media for manipulating the narrative. I was grateful that the media attention was keeping the issue at the front of the political agenda – and knew that this was the best opportunity for change we would ever get – but was grieved by how it distorted the storyline.

❖❖❖

Journalists are informed by a code of practice that includes reporting the truth, minimising harm, acting independently, and being both accountable and transparent.[8] Yet, there are times when people in the media struggle with the competing pressures of telling the truth, grabbing public attention, and selling a story. The term 'fake news', referring to the dissemination of potentially harmful misinformation, became popularised in contemporary language thanks to Donald Trump's efforts in the 2016 presidential election. It became so influential that school courses were developed to teach children strategies to detect it. 'Fake news' was voted 'word of the decade' in a 2021 *Macquarie Dictionary* poll.[9]

There are strategies such as 'gotcha' journalism, where a journalist hammers an interviewee with the same questions until they finally get muddled and incriminate themselves. Looking back, perhaps there were elements of this in some of the interviews with Leesa Vlahos.

This might be the hard edge of investigative journalism. But it may also result in the dehumanisation of the subject, seeing them as grist for the mill, rather than as a person who may have a complex story behind the presenting issue.

This type of journalism is not unlike the process of 'othering' that can undermine healthcare practitioners' relationships. The media narrative – and therefore the public perception – involved the 'othering' of the Oakden staff. A group was created, and certain characteristics were assigned to all those perceived as belonging to that group. The narrative was more accessible when all staff were seen as harmful and abusive. The Oakden story needed telling, but the dominant public narrative did not do justice to the truth.

❖ ❖ ❖

Returning to the political landscape, the 2018 state election came just weeks after the release of the ICAC Report. The Commissioner's sentiment regarding South Australia's shame was echoed in rapid-fire television advertisements authorised by the opposition – who, by this stage, seemed almost certain to form the next government. The opposition's advertising did not hold back in its appraisal of premier Jay Weatherill and his government.

'Damned, disgrace; shameful, failure,' one campaign ad commenced. 'How could Labor let the horrors of Oakden happen? No, Jay, it's not okay!'[10]

It is a fact of life that every political party pulls the rhetorical stop out in the context of an election fight – and Oakden was a prime target. What these advertisements did, of course, was contribute to the overarching public perception of the story, played out online, on radio, on TV, and in print.

In the months after the opposition was elected, we went through our first, highly scrutinised, high-pressure accreditation at Northgate House. The service was now under national hospital and health service accreditation standards, rather than the Commonwealth aged care standards that had applied to the service at Oakden. The threat of punitive action if we were not successful loomed menacingly, and there were whispers of people losing their jobs should there be any recommendations or unmet standards. I do not believe that would – or could – have happened, but the fact that people were talking that way reflected the anxious tone of the times.

We made it through the scrutiny, with accreditors moved to tears by the stories of transformation beginning to emerge from the families of people who had transitioned from Oakden to Northgate House. We received commendations rather than recommendations, greeted by a universal, organisational sigh of relief. A story of recovery was underway.

Following our accreditation success, the new minister for Health and Wellbeing (which included the mental health portfolio), Stephen Wade, held a press conference at Northgate House to assure the public that progress was being made. We gathered outside with the media, and the minister spoke briefly, acknowledging our success and making a commitment to the reform agenda.

When it was my turn, I also made a brief statement: 'This is a line-in-the-sand moment,' I told the reporters, 'although we know we still have a long way to go.'

With remarkable predictability, and despite the positive nature of the occasion, the usual questions were asked all over again.

'How many staff here also worked at Oakden?'

'How are you monitoring them?'

We had been through tough times. But by this time, I knew that we were turning things around. Our team was increasingly committed, including staff who had transitioned across from Oakden, among whom were some remarkable people.

I'd had enough of the repetitive line of questioning and, for better or worse, I bit back at the reporter.

'Yes, there are staff working here who worked at Oakden, and they are excellent. We are very proud of all our staff.' I had paid a penny, so I went in for a pound.

'As the media,' I lectured, 'you have responsibility to the public in terms of the narrative you create. To suggest that the staff who worked at Oakden were all "bad nurses" is highly irresponsible. It's just not true. You need to think about the impact of the story you're telling. There were very caring staff who worked at Oakden, against the odds, and now they're part of our learning, growing team here – and we're proud of them.'[11]

Unknown to me, the interview was being streamed online by one of the networks present. Our team was inside, watching it play out – many still wounded by the events of the preceding year. Hearing themselves being publicly and passionately defended became a turning point for us all. In that moment I earned a new level of trust. Together, we began to turn the tables on the burdensome legacy we carried.

Also participating in the press conference were relatives of residents who had made the journey from Oakden to Northgate House. Their voices were the most prominent and influential of the day. In contrast to the stories from the families who had become the public faces of Oakden, stories that remained historical due to the death of their loved family members at Oakden prior to its closure, these voices offered hope rather than tragedy.

For the first time, there was a headline that sparked optimism: 'Northgate aged-care centre gets top gong.'[12]

The typical errors in detail notwithstanding, finally there was the hope of a different narrative. Most importantly, there was a shift in the story we told ourselves.

13

What matters most

What went wrong at Oakden, and what so often goes wrong in health systems, schools, politics and communities, is a loss of connection with people and their stories – of their uniqueness and value. It is too easy to stop seeing people as being like us and make them other than ourselves, reducing their identity to illness, to a difference of opinion or a divergence of culture. We are frequently uncomfortable sitting with variance and struggle to find common ground. This discomfort with difference, and the tendency toward othering, underpinned the degradation and dehumanisation we saw at the Oakden Campus. It fuelled the political, punitive and reactionary blame culture that followed the exposure of what had happened.

'There but for the grace of God ...' said Helen, a senior psychiatry colleague we brought in from interstate during the early reform period.

We were managing the hundreds of complaints that had emerged alongside the avalanche of media reports. Helen came to help review some of the most challenging cases. With many years of experience running older persons' mental health services, she knew shades of Oakden could be found everywhere. Sure, Oakden was a particular example, but similar cultural problems occur to some measure in many settings. Just hang out in health and aged care services – or any number of other enterprises – for a while, and you will encounter them. We should be cautious about passing too harsh and hasty a judgement on Oakden. Helen understood this, acknowledging: 'It could have been us.'

What matters most

If we want to do better, we need to get back to basics. Our business must be about people. We need to find the story behind the person. We need to cultivate respectful ways of dealing with difference and disagreement. We need to make space for people to be themselves when, for whatever reason, they look, believe, vote, speak and behave differently from us. We can choose compassion, courtesy and kindness and ensure that we don't lose sight of the personhood of others.

One experience, more than any other, brought this home for me in the challenging months after the Oakden Report. We had moved everyone out of Oakden. Our team continued to support the residential aged care providers who had offered permanent homes to former residents, most with great success and a few with challenges that required scaffolding. Nonetheless, the transition took place successfully.

We had moved the smaller group of residents who still needed specialist care to our new service at Northgate, where we were embarking on our journey toward a transformed culture. A decommissioning process at the Oakden Campus began, unpacking the years of institutional clutter that had mounted up in every cupboard and corner.

One of the residents we moved across to Northgate House was an older Hungarian woman called Lily. She was diminutive, but she had a fiery passion which, despite living with dementia, would emerge in her efforts to communicate and connect. Lily had lived through the Second World War in Europe. She had experienced the deprivation and trauma of living under German occupation and the subsequent ascendency of Soviet control. Uncertainty and anxiety had been dominant themes during this period of her life and during a challenging journey of migration to establish a new life on the other side of the world. It should not have been a surprise when the consequences of trauma and anxiety surfaced as part of Lily's experience of dementia.

Lily had lost her English language skills, and efforts to communicate in her native Hungarian through an interpreter were mostly incoherent. She struggled with people providing her hygiene care, and when confronted with moments of exposure and discomfort, responded with efforts to defend herself. Residential aged care providers were unable to manage these challenging moments. Consequently, Lily found herself living at Oakden and was among the very first residents at Northgate House. Lily's family had been anxious about the day she might return to mainstream aged care, fearful that she could not be properly cared for in that environment.

A short while after her transfer to Northgate House, Lily took a turn for the worse. Her physical health rapidly deteriorated, and it became evident that she was reaching the end of her life. Given the context of all that had happened, it would have been inappropriate to transfer her elsewhere, so she became the first person to receive palliative care in the new unit. We called for support from our local community palliative-care team, and the nursing staff at Northgate House worked hard to provide a comfortable environment for Lily and her family.

My one frustration was a lack of personal belongings that honoured Lily's life history, and which would have made for a truly personalised environment. Neither our team nor Lily's children or grandchildren could find any items that captured the essence of her story.

After a short period of palliative care, Lily slipped beyond life. Her family were concurrently grief-stricken and relieved. The aftermath of her death – deemed a 'death in custody' because of Lily's status under the *Guardianship and Administration Act* – included mandatory reporting to the coroner's office. Because of our shameful recent past, the coroner had declared a public interest in thoroughly examining every death associated with Oakden. This was necessary, but it added to the stress experienced by Lily's family.

The day after Lily's death, I was back at the Oakden Campus. For whatever reason, I opened the door to one of the many rooms I had not entered before. It was an old patient bay converted into a storeroom. Industrial shelves lined the walls and were heavily laden with boxes and suitcases. Junk had been jammed into the centre of the room, including broken wheelchairs, tables, beds and trunks. It was hard to make a path through it all, and as I pushed past an old mattress, I noticed old faecal matter caked and dried along its surface. I cringed.

I opened the first suitcase I came to and caught my breath. It was Lily's.

She had died the night before, cared for as best we could, but without being surrounded by precious details from her life. Now I found myself holding black-and-white photographs of Lily, and an insight into her story. There was Lily on her wedding day, looking joyful next to her new husband. There was a photograph of her holding her baby, and others with her family as they grew up and became increasingly Australian.

There were personal papers, under which I found items of jewellery, a pendant on a chain and a simple, small ring, the metal dimmed by time and dirt but with a modest, gleaming gemstone. Looking up at me from within the suitcase was a woman who had lived, and loved, and danced, and wept.

For a moment I stood and held the items in silence, staring at them while the room seemed to swirl around me. I struggled to process the fact that these items, which told the story of Lily's life and relationships, had been boxed up in a cupboard filled with broken equipment and dirty mattresses – that they had not enriched her environment, nor had communicated who she was to the people providing care for her as she died. Who had made the decision that they should be taken away and put here? What did this say about how she was seen and known?

I surveyed the room and realised there were other suitcases, and boxes, similarly filled with clothing, photographs and personal items; pieces of the lives and memories of people whose journeys had ended at Oakden, piled up on shelves.

The emotional impact of the preceding months contracted into that moment for me. Standing in a storeroom, holding a ring and a photograph of a wedding, precious moments of life overlooked and left behind.

I cried.

I grieved for Lily. I grieved for us all and how we had failed. We had allowed a system to lose the person and box up their story, almost as if they had never lived.

My experience of finding the boxed lives of former residents is not unique. In their moving book, *The Lives They Left Behind*, Darby Penney and Peter Stastny documented the stories of ten lifelong residents of the Willard State Psychiatric Hospital in New York, following the discovery of 427 suitcases interred in the hospital attic. The suitcases were discovered by two local women and a visiting historian during the period of the institution's decommissioning and demolition in the 1980s and 1990s.

Penny and Stastny described the finding:

Once the door was pried open, they were struck by an awesome sight: a beam of sunlight streaming down a central corridor that separated rows of wooden racks tightly filled with suitcases of all shapes and sizes – men's on the left side, women's on the right, alphabetised, labelled, and covered by layers of bird droppings, apparently untouched for a great many years.

Crates, trunks, hundreds of standard suitcases, doctors' bags and many-shaped containers were all neatly arrayed under the watchful eyes of the pigeons who had come to join the lost souls, and their worldly possessions … This upper room exuded an unearthly air, a hovering presence of hundreds of souls or spirits attached to the many people who had handled and worn the items in those bags before they were packed, who had read the books, written in the diaries, and looked into the mirrors they contained.[1]

Historically, it is a feature of the experience of many people with mental illness, disability, and dementia that they are pathologised – that they are seen primarily through the lens of their diagnosis. In this way, they are marginalised and dehumanised – made 'other'.

Penney and Stastny described what motivated them to write their book. They lamented that 'these individuals never had the chance to tell their stories outside of the confines of psychiatry'. They went on:

What might be revealed by comparing the personal artefacts from their pre-institutional lives with the way they were perceived by doctors and hospital staff? Regardless of what might have troubled them, we were struck by the sundering of who they were as people from who they became as mental patients.[2]

Confronted by the chaotic library of Oakden residents' lives, I encountered this same phenomenon.

I called Jackie Hanson, the CEO, and explained what I had found. She cried.

An inventory of all the items was made, and a process of open disclosure undertaken. Most of the belongings were returned to families, with some donated to charity at their request. With a renewed commitment, we vowed to remember the person at the centre of care. It is a fragile and easily forgotten commitment, not least in the face of financial and service-flow pressures. But we must recognise and resist our tendencies towards othering and pathologising.

And here lies the most critical lesson from Oakden: what matters most are people. How we treat people and how we make them feel. Whatever field we labour in, whatever position we hold, whoever we are – the way we treat the people we serve, and those we serve with, matters. The Oakden story is a composite volume of interacting narratives across public, political, media, staff, family, and personal domains. It is a story of failure, but it offers an opportunity for a new narrative of reinvention and learning – if we turn our attention to what matters most.

PART 3

Finding Our Way Back

14

Co-design and compassion

'Nothing about us without us!' J.I. Charlton, 1998[1]

James Charlton's declaration reverberates with advocacy and activism; daring and defiance. Emerging from the disability rights movement and taken up by other marginalised communities, including many people living with dementia, it is an assertion of the human right to have agency over our own lives and to be present with equal voice in our communities, able to tell our stories and speak for ourselves. One of the messages that hit home during the immediate period after the Oakden Report was that the voices, stories and priorities of people with experience of what it was like to live at Oakden needed to inform and guide system redesign. This principle is relevant in many settings.

After the Oakden Report, an oversight committee was formed, bringing together key people from across South Australia with skills, insight and independence – including people with experience of being on the receiving end of our services. Their job was to offer wisdom, speak freely, and ask tough questions to ensure that the reform process stayed on track. As the Head of Unit, brought in to provide clinical leadership of the redesign, I attended the committee meetings reporting on the work that was going on. The committee members were encouraging, cheering on our change-team, while probing in such a way as to not let any issues slip by.

Also reporting to the oversight committee were six co-design teams, each focused on one of the six recommendations of the Oakden Report. The idea of co-design is important here. It refers to including everyone who will use a service, product or change in practice, as equal partners through the entire process of design and decision-making. It still requires design expertise and doesn't negate the need for governance and accountability – but it does reflect a commitment to doing things *with* the people most affected by a change, not just *for* them.[2] People with experience of having a family member at Oakden were invited to join every co-design team, alongside clinicians, industry representatives and service planners. Courageous people took up these opportunities, unafraid to speak up and remind the clinicians and departmental executives of promises that had been made.

The teams got busy, developing blueprints for what system redesign might look like. They invited input from people from across the community. Requests for written feedback on documents and communiqués were distributed widely, resulting in a plethora of letters and emails.

Invitations to a series of 'gallery walks' were sent out, welcoming the community to open discussions. Gallery walk sessions commenced with morning or afternoon tea, followed by storytelling from family members of people who had lived at Oakden, then a report about where progress was being made. Participants would stroll around a series of 'ideas stations', which presented information about proposed reforms. There would be a facilitator standing by each station to answer questions. People could provide input, or react to the ideas presented, indicating support or disagreement by peppering posters at the stations with green or red paper dots.

From these conversations, the co-design teams proposed new models of care. Ideas about new types of buildings and environments emerged. The teams recommended governance principles that would give the community confidence that the terrible failings of Oakden would not be repeated. Despite the concurrent stress, system reactivity and sheer hard work, it was an agile time in which rumblings of reinvention stirred. We were all hopeful that real change could be achieved.

The outputs of all this hard work of discussing, dreaming and designing were published as a weighty document in June 2018.[3] Like the

Oakden Report over a year earlier, the recommendations and blueprints offered were accepted and endorsed by the South Australian Government and the Department of Health.[4] It marked the completion of a first phase of redesign. It also presented a new challenge: to what extent would well-intentioned plans be translated into real-world action?

❖❖❖

Recognising that it's impossible to separate culture from care – one leads to the other – the most fundamental finding of the Oakden Report was the profound failure in organisational culture, resulting in the loss of dignity and humanity for everyone involved, residents, families and staff. My view is that without addressing the issue of culture – which tackles both heart and behaviour – the best models of care and finest buildings remain hollow.

To address this, one of the dedicated and enthusiastic co-design teams focused in on the report's recommendation for intentional culture reform as a foundation for all the other reform work. This co-design team was chaired by Jackie Hanson and included Barb Spriggs, whose tenacious storytelling had blown the lid on Oakden. I was one of the clinicians on the team. Two facilitators supported the co-design process and the team commenced zealous deliberations on what change should look like. We asked the questions: 'How do we heal healthcare culture when it is sick?' And: 'What should our culture be?'

Through discussion, productive argument, analysing data, formulating themes and refining ideas, the co-design team developed the *culture framework*.[5] It was a blueprint that set out a guiding philosophy for our future services, and provided four actionable priorities that the team believed would help us get where we needed to be.

There was one word more than any other that came up in the discussions of the co-design team and in the feedback from members of the public: *compassion*. Everyone agreed that being compassionate and delivering compassionate care must be the cornerstone of reform.

The origin of the word compassion, from Latin, literally means '*to suffer with another*'.[6] The co-design team aspired to a system of care, filled with people who would see and be moved by the suffering of others, and who would be motivated to action, coming alongside those who suffer to offer help and hope.[7]

The team also mulled over recurrent ideas that brought attention to the relationships between the person, their family, and the people providing their care – and how healthy partnerships are essential to humane systems of care.

In his book *Dementia Reconsidered: The Person Comes First*, Tom Kitwood defined *personhood* as 'the standing or status bestowed upon one human being by others in the context of a relationship and social being. It implies recognition, respect and trust'.[8] This is an important definition. It presents an antithesis to the phenomenon of *othering* that I have referred to repeatedly within this text – and that was a prominent cultural occurrence at Oakden – where personhood was denied and lost. Kitwood's definition places identity, dignity and effective care in the context of relationships.

Drawing these ideas together, the co-design team referred to the UK Leadership in Compassionate Care program, which connected *relationship-centred care* with the translation of compassion into everyday practice.[9] This program advocated that quality healthcare requires respectful relationships, based on empathy, that motivate the people providing care to actively understand and relieve distress and suffering. These relationships rely upon knowledge of the person and their family, and a commitment to work *with* them – not just *for* or *on* them – to support people making decisions about their own lives in the best way they possibly can.

And so, the co-design team agreed that *compassionate relationship-centred care* should be the philosophical foundation of the culture framework, and the guiding principle for everything we aimed to deliver to people from then on. To achieve this, the team asserted, we would need to prioritise four actions.

The first of these was to *build a values-based workforce*. Time and effort should be put into thinking about, defining and sharing the core values that support compassionate, relationship-centred care – values such as empathy, kindness, patience and respect. The team set the challenge of ensuring that values were translated into action. There is no point for an organisation to put forward a set of aspirational, humane values if people at all levels do not 'walk the talk'.

To build a values-based workforce, the team argued that recruitment should prioritise character and values, rather than just looking at skills and qualifications, or falling into the trap of many vacancy-carrying health services of looking for the best available 'warm body' to plug a hole in the workforce.

Values-based recruitment reduces staff turnover and sick leave, improves morale, increases job satisfaction, and enhances care.[10] It requires creativity, but there are all sorts of tools that can help: problem-based scenarios, group interview sessions, and values-based psychometric testing.[11] The co-design team also called for a commitment that every recruitment panel would always include a person who had received care from the service – or a family member – to help decide who would join the care team.

Later on, when we were putting the priorities of the culture framework into practice, we introduced role-play and storytelling to interviews. Sometimes, we would ask the person being interviewed to answer a question as if they were the person receiving care. In other questions we would show pictures of older people in different situations – images that depicted isolation, cultural issues, questions about using medications, or the importance of community for older people. We would ask the person being interviewed to tell us a story about what might have been happening in the image, and to tell us how that made them feel. There were many profound and moving moments as people opened up with stories about themselves and the older people they loved. We learnt about people's lives and grandparents, their fears of getting older themselves. On some occasions, the person and those on the panel found themselves in tears. We came to better understand what was really important to people hoping to work with our team, giving us a sense of how they might be a good fit.

The co-design team turned to a second priority: *cultivating psychological safety*. As described earlier, psychological safety refers to a work environment where team members feel safe to voice ideas, to provide and seek candid feedback, to collaborate with others and experiment.[12] It frees people from not feeling able to bring their whole-selves to work – and therefore acknowledging their weakness and need for growth. Psychological safety creates more courageous and creative workplaces. It encourages a generous contribution of ideas from team members to a shared enterprise.

Many health systems have limited psychological safety. Staff are often highly anxious about making a mistake and getting in trouble for it – and this promotes covering up. This was exactly how things were at Oakden, and in the difficult early days after the publication of the report. The co-design team wanted to change this.

Psychological safety makes it safe to admit and learn from our errors. It facilitates speaking up within systems, so problems don't remain hidden. It is an essential condition if we hope to foster innovation, which requires us to be safe enough to have a go at new things. It provides rich soil for learning and growth.

Balancing the first two priorities, the co-design team described a third: *facilitating excellence in care*. They advocated for investment in adequately resourced staffing profiles – clearly identified as a problem at Oakden and with implications elsewhere in Commonwealth-funded aged care. They recognised the necessary investment in research and practice focused on dementia and older peoples' mental health. They called for targeted education and qualifications, which, in our case, related to helping staff deeply understand the mental health and wellbeing needs of older people. They challenged workplaces to create new opportunities and career pathways to foster staff growth, and argued for support of 'ground-up' rather than 'top-down' approaches to quality and safety activities. The premise for all this was that unless people are personally engaged and have ownership of what they are doing, the outcomes will fall short of true excellence.

Co-design and compassion

The co-design team established a fourth and final priority that could be summed up with a simple statement: *We are open and honest.*

The co-design team referred to Francis' recommendations in the Mid Staffordshire Report. Francis described health service executives' and managers' responsibility to provide absolute transparency and candour.[13] Along similar lines, the Oakden Report had identified failures in clinical and corporate governance, and a culture of secrecy and rhetorical subterfuge. By contrast, the co-design team called for everyone to be completely honest and upfront about the business of providing care – from the cleaners to the CEO. There was the expectation that any health and social care service, and the people running it, should be held accountable to deliver against all the values, standards and behaviours required to provide people with compassionate, relationship-centred care.

In practical terms, the team considered that this should involve reliable mechanisms for managing complaints, providing feedback, and being open about issues when something goes wrong. It would mean people who use services should be included in governance and decision-making processes. It would mean a commitment to not keeping secrets or inhibiting the flow of information. There should be no cover-ups, no political spin, just truthfulness.

The co-design team brought together designers, with people from the community, and clinicians who aspired to *be* and *do* better. It championed the voice of people who had lived through Oakden, and who urged 'nothing about us, without us!'. It illustrated the productive power of partnership. As a result of collaboration, the *culture framework* provided a song sheet with compassionate human relationships as its focus. It offered a more trustworthy future – if we could take it off the page and turn it into music.

15

The Culture Club

I consider my meeting with Andrew Stevens serendipitous because, had it been left up to me, it wouldn't have happened. Andrew and his colleague Diana Renner had left their secure jobs, Andrew as head of the Executive Education programs at Adelaide University, and Diana as a lawyer. They established the consultancy firm Uncharted Leadership Institute, using their collective years of learning and reflection to help other enterprises and individuals develop courageous leadership and positive organisational cultures.

Andrew took an idea to the Executive Director of System Leadership and Design in the South Australian Department of Health. He pointed out that the typical way in which health systems – indeed, many businesses in general – develop their workforce is to look for 'bright young things', people with evident potential. They invest in sending these emerging leaders away to courses and development programs, usually at significant expense. Andrew's idea was to pilot a program where, rather than taking a few people out of the workplace to engage in learning and leadership growth, everyone's opportunity to grow would be brought into the workplace and would ultimately become the usual way of doing business.

Andrew's proposal was heavily influenced by the work of Robert Kegan, Lisa Lahey and their associates at the Harvard Business School. In their 2016 book, *An Everyone Culture*, they described an approach to work they called the 'Deliberately Developmental Organisation'

(DDO).[1] They pointed out that, in most workplaces, we tend to be doing a second job that no one is paying us for – covering up the things we are not good at; hiding our personal life and our vulnerabilities. They provided insight into organisations that have modelled a different way of working by redefining their core values, creating safety for robust communication from the ground up, promoting every person's growth, and holding everyone to account for their contribution. When I first encountered these ideas, I recognised their coherence with our co-designed culture framework's four priorities. Kegan's and Lahey's work became such an important part of what we learnt as a team that I've even made a respectful reference to them in the title of this book.

But when Jackie Hanson nominated Northgate House as the site for the proposed pilot project, I was cautious. We were still going through so much change. The Oakden Campus had closed months before. Northgate House was evolving, and we had blitzed our first accreditation. But workplace trauma simmered. Staff remained distrustful of senior leadership. They carried the historical burden of being misunderstood and harshly judged. Given this, I was not confident that we were ready for what Andrew and his team were offering.

When we're unsure ourselves, it can be the wisdom of others that results in valuable change. Both Jackie Hanson and the Chief Executive decided that Northgate House was the ideal site for the project. And so it was that I learnt we would be embarking on an expedition of discovery. I had no inkling of the extent to which this experience, or the relationships and conversations it entailed, would bring together the threads of learning percolating in me throughout my time at Oakden.

❖ ❖ ❖

Staff gathered to launch our project over afternoon tea with CEO Jackie Hanson, Andrew Stevens, and visitors from the Department of Health. It felt strange and surreal. The atmosphere was tense; these people were not at ease with each other. No one knew what to expect. Everyone was fumblingly polite.

We made small talk about the weather and drank our tea. The staff and visitors sat in a circle beneath the Northgate House veranda, looking at each other in anticipation. I thanked everyone for being there, confirmed that we would be commencing the pilot project to build our team, and handed over to Jackie to get started.

Jackie then made a courageous and counter-cultural move for a CEO.

She apologised.

'It's been a difficult time, and a lot has happened,' she said. 'I made decisions very quickly and did what I felt I had to do at the time. I was trying to protect the vulnerable people living at Oakden, but in doing that, I took some punitive decisions. I recognise that some of those decisions caused distress and harm to you. I appreciate that it's not okay. I know we all need to learn from this and do better.'

Jackie had also been going through a process of learning and change. Feisty in temperament, her baseline approach to any exchange had been assertiveness. Many staff were afraid of her. She was serious about governance and keen to run a tight ship, but her engagement with the workforce had been hampered by an appearance of severity.

I had the opportunity to work with Jackie in a way that few other people did, and I saw a different side of her. We forged a bond that can only result from living through the same hard times. I witnessed how she changed, driven by the scandal's intense pressure and political context – which wore her down. More importantly, Jackie listened to hundreds of stories from family members of Oakden residents. That listening transformed her.

She also connected with the experiences of people who worked in the service. Both groups had been neglected. Both groups had been seen as low in value. Both were victims of being seen as 'other'. Jackie gained insight into how the lack of psychological safety in health services impacts the people who work within those systems and how readily staff can be pushed into an anxiety zone, causing defensiveness. Flawed and faltering, she began to change as a leader.

So, it was a decisive moment when she sat with the group of staff that afternoon and opened our new venture with an apology. It did not undo all the damage – no one expected things to be immediately changed – but it did give hope. Jackie modelled an aspect of courageous leadership that is a prerequisite to changing workplace culture. She demonstrated vulnerability. She made it okay to fail, to get things wrong and to apologise with transparency. We had a long way to go, but we couldn't have had a more fitting start to the project.

❖❖❖

Andrew and the team from Uncharted Leadership proposed a three-phase strategy for the project. Phase one would focus on communication, team building and psychological safety. Phase two would involve connecting team members with their areas for growth – not so much relating to their clinical or technical skills, but their personal development. Phase three would support the team in becoming self-sustaining in whatever we found worked and wanted to keep. From that point, the external support could be withdrawn, and we would go it alone.

There was an early (and somewhat unrealistic) expectation that phase one would take six to eight weeks. But that's not how culture-change projects like this work. Unsurprisingly, it took much longer – it was more than nine months before we were ready to move to phase two. One of the gifts that Andrew and his team gave us was that they stayed with us, flexibly adjusting the plan and the goals as we went, learning alongside us, long after the grant they had received from the Department of Health dried up.

After that initial meeting with Jackie Hanson over afternoon tea, we started meeting weekly, inviting everyone in the team. One challenge with a program like this in a 24/7 clinical service was making it accessible to all. Meeting with everyone at any one time was impossible, as clinical staff were needed on the floor. Most team members worked different shifts, including nights, and it took weeks to give everyone an opportunity to attend a meeting. In this context, it was challenging to build momentum across the team. Nevertheless, we pushed ahead, believing that at least starting conversations with some of the team members was better than not having them at all.

Our early meetings were clunky. The same people talked each week, me among them. Others said nothing. Andrew and his team facilitated conversations by breaking us into smaller groups, gently helping us to revisit some of the trauma. Gradually, people warmed up.

Not everyone was on board. One team member, who was extraordinarily diligent but very traditional, came to me one day, saying: 'I can't see the point of all these conversations we're having about how we get along with each other. It's a waste of time – and our taxes are paying for it. We should all be out on the floor, working and delivering care.'

I was taken aback but needed to reflect on the criticism. I realised that certain conversations in the workplace were never disputed. Clinical handover, for instance, is an essential element of communication in any health service. We commit time and resources to ensure this occurs and use proformas to ensure that specific quality standards are met. But I also knew that the other conversations we were now having were just as meaningful. I became convinced that quarantining time and putting effort into conversations about *how* we work together, not only about *what* we do, were just as critical. The relationships and safety cultivated by these conversations promised better clinical and task-related working as an outcome.

Andrew introduced us to the practice of the 'check-in' and 'check-out' and, by repeating this each week, a transformation began to take place in the team. It was a simple process. Every time we came together for a meeting, we started by checking in. The practice involved each person having the opportunity to say their name, acknowledge that they were checking in, and then talk about whatever was most pressing for them. The process recognised that everyone came to that moment with various thoughts, pressures and issues crowding their minds. Some people were just starting a shift, having come from their busy home lives. Others were coming from their morning shift with incomplete checklists hanging over them. All of us had matters that could distract us from the work we needed to do together. All of us were at risk of covering up what was really happening on the inside – which could impact how we entered that moment of shared enterprise.

'It's Bernice,' someone might say, 'and I'm checking in. I've just come from dropping the kids at daycare, and I'm frazzled because they were crying the whole way in the car. I'm stressed about leaving them there.'

It was a simple strategy that created a space to experiment with bridging the perceived gap between the 'work' and 'home' versions of ourselves. Cautiously, people started to open up and let others know more about themselves. It was imperfect, but it felt real. The check-out was a reverse process. It allowed people to briefly reflect on the meeting's content, bring closure to the work, and shift gears to whatever was coming next for them – going home, hitting the floor to provide clinical care, or getting on with other business.

As we reinforced the habit of checking in and out, week after week, the team changed. The practice spread to handovers and governance meetings, which soon became more personal interactions. I learnt the importance of simple, meaningful, accessible and repeatable practices. I started to think of our check-ins and other practices we developed as 'rituals'. They supported sustainability by being built into normal routines, while connecting us with the reason for doing them – just like lighting a candle in a church might remind a person of an underlying spiritual truth. Every time we checked in with each other, we were actively doing something that reminded us that we wanted to reduce power imbalances in our team, that we all needed each other, and that we could build the culture together by being courageous enough to bring our whole selves to work.

Sometimes our check-ins were brief and appeared superficial. Sometimes, they offered us insights into our colleagues that we would otherwise have been unlikely to gain. One day, one of our nurses, who was sharp as a whip, superefficient and always immaculately groomed, announced: 'I'm Diva, checking in. I'm really looking forward to getting home from work today because, for the first time in my life, I'm going to have a lesson to learn how to ride a bike.'

Everyone laughed. We had got to know Diva a little better: she was no longer just an impressive clinical logistician; she was a human with a life to live and lessons to learn.

After practising this 'ritual' for a while, we started having remarkable moments where our checking in and out became emotional and therapeutic. The work we do with people living with dementia can be difficult; it can take a toll on team members – many of whom had family members with dementia, making the work even more personal. After one session, in which we had debriefed following the death of a resident, one of the nurses, Bronnie, checked out by reflecting on how our work kept her connected to her mother, whom she had nursed through dementia to the end-of-life just a couple of years earlier. 'Understanding what we do for people is so important,' she said through tears. We were all moved. Her check-out grounded us back in the things that matter most.

As these meetings took on a life of their own, we renamed them: reflecting the high prevalence of children of the eighties in our team, and several Boy George fans, we started referring to our meetings as 'The Culture Club'. It stuck. I even received a classic CD by the iconic British band from my Secret Santa at our team Christmas function that year.

Having everyone attend the Culture Club was revelatory. We had nurses, both registered and enrolled. We had allied health practitioners: occupational therapist, social worker, physiotherapist, speech pathologist, pharmacist. We had admin and hotel services staff – the people who answer the phone, welcome visitors, clean the unit and prepare the food. Our meetings deliberately brought everyone together on the premise that we left our rank and roles at the door. Everyone had the same right to speak and be heard.

It is not an everyday occurrence in health services for doctors to sit down with hotel services team members. But it changed my life as the senior doctor for the service – a position of traditional power and privilege – to learn to listen to members of the cleaning team. I learnt so much from them, about our residents, about the team's climate, about what was required to make the service more effective. I was often impressed and humbled by the creativity, wisdom and insight of this team of people who received a fraction of my overblown salary yet brought so much love and commitment to their work. It's very difficult to deconstruct differences in power that are so easily established within hierarchical organisations. My experience was that learning to listen and build relationships through sincere conversation was a life-changing, countercultural experience.

A couple of the cleaning staff, Nicola and Kath, became influential culture-change leaders. They continued to do their regular work but contributed ideas and innovation to the unit, which they would not normally have had permission to do. They contributed ideas about workflow, environmental improvements, and insightful observations about what worked well for residents. Nicola was keen on sewing and one day came to work with a prototype of a beautiful floral chair cover she had created for one of the resident's chairs. There was no doubt that this was beyond the call of duty.

Part way through phase one of the Growth Culture project, Andrew and his colleagues organised a workshop to examine the concept of psychological safety in greater detail. One of the facilitators took us through related concepts, making a list on a giant Post-it note as we went. After some reflection, Kay, one of our hotel services team, spoke up: 'I truly believe that we're doing much of this,' she said. 'We weren't – even three months ago,' she went on, 'but now we are. We're changing.'

Some weeks later, we evaluated our progress. Nicola, speaking on behalf of the hotel services team, said: 'We always had things to say. What changed for us is that we were given a voice.'

We thought it would be helpful for the team to articulate a statement of shared values and vision. This is, after all, what teams tend to do. We wanted it to be something that would resonate with the whole team, capture our purpose, and motivate us toward growth.

We put our heads together and quickly encountered difficulty. The daunting challenge, which would need to be reflected in our statement, was not in starting out with good intentions but in following through to translatable action. We were stuck. The trauma of failure and shame had caused deep wounds in the team's identity and, despite our progress as a service, we could not capture a positive vision in words. Thinking on his feet, Andrew suggested we circle back and talk about all the things the media had said about Oakden over the previous year and how they had impacted the team.

Research indicates that in both personal relationships and in the workplace, the ratio of positive to negative feedback required to ensure growth is about 5:1.[2] For most people, we need five positive comments for every single criticism to remain motivated and be encouraged to grow. This has impact on whether a team is high or low performing. A barrage of continual criticism and negativity does not help people perform at their best.

Reflecting on the stories told in the media, by the government and within our health network, it was no surprise that the mud had stuck in ways that had not yet been resolved. A self-narrative was deeply embedded within the team. Revisiting the news headlines became a therapeutic process. People acknowledged how difficult it had been. Staff who had worked at Oakden acknowledged that they believed they could never get another job, that they would never be able to leave the reputation behind.

Rather than leaving us there, Andrew turned our attention toward the future.

'But what about in two years?' he asked. 'When the media come back, what do we want them to say about this team – about Northgate House?'

There was a pause while everyone reflected. Then the floodgates opened:

'Best older persons' mental health service in Adelaide.'

'Northgate House delivers outstanding care.'

'Everyone comes home at Northgate House.'

People laughed as they proposed the headlines, enjoying the irony of the contrast.

This activity took several weeks. We opened an online survey asking everyone to contribute and voted on the most resonant headlines. It was both fun and healing. The positive phrases themselves were encouraging and affected the tone of the team. We started tipping the balance back in favour of positivity and hope.

Having collected data from the exercise, the team reconvened for the Culture Club. We displayed the most popular headlines and comments on a board and started brainstorming, seeking to agree on the keywords.

'It's all about compassion,' someone said.

There was strong agreement, and we drew a circle around it on the list.

'I think it's about providing exceptional person-centred care,' said someone else.

'Acceptance,' said another, 'and kindness and respect.'

'We try things out – things that other people might not do,' someone volunteered. 'That's why I think innovation is a keyword.'

The conversation became a glowing list of hopefulness in front of us.

'Teamwork,' someone pointed out with gravity. 'The most important thing we've learnt so far is that we must be a team. We can't do our work if we don't do it together. Everyone here matters.'

'Yes, being a team makes it easier to come to work,' someone else chimed in.

I was excited to be experiencing such a climate of change. It was evident that the work we were doing was paying off. Others felt it too, and the enthusiasm built.

We thinned the list down to just a few words and started putting them together as a statement. I love words and could have manipulated the exercise to craft a statement, but I didn't need to. The spontaneous enthusiasm of the group carried it along. A resonant message emerged from this process, and we all agreed that we'd found the statement we wanted to be our headline:

At Northgate House, we deliver exceptional, innovative and compassionate person and family-centred care through teamwork, where everyone matters; everyone contributes; everyone grows.

'Teamwork' was the pivotal word, around which the whole statement made sense. And the statement was owned by the team – not just the leadership team, nor the executive or Andrew, or the Department of Health's facilitators, as supportive as they were. The principle of co-design was again at play here, just as it was in developing the culture framework. Things are better when people get to create them for themselves. There was a story unfolding at Northgate House. What had happened at Oakden was not the final chapter for this group of people, and they realised they had a chance of being co-authors of what happened next.

16

Telling our stories

'Everyone matters, everyone contributes, everyone grows ...' The phrase became a rallying cry. But we still faced the challenge of embedding change sustainably, so that we would not become an example of a superficial, temporary modification of behaviour that would return to baseline as soon as attention turned elsewhere.

'Our culture will be the result of things we do either by *default* or by *design*,' I'd say to the team. 'That's why we always need to be *deliberate*.'

Before progressing with the project's second phase, the leadership team asked everyone to vote on whether to continue. We knew that most of the team was on board, but some team members still struggled to trust anything the organisation did. We wanted to give them a chance to air their concerns – to make their voices heard.

The result of the vote was not unanimous, but it was nevertheless a robust, democratic, 'Yes, let's keep going.'

We started talking about Personal Improvement Goals – 'PIGs' for short. We weren't talking about becoming more proficient in technical skills, such as delivering a particular clinical practice. We were talking about the opportunity for personal growth and what might get in the way of achieving this. Several team members spoke about their difficulty communicating their thoughts and ideas in a team setting. Others talked about struggling to manage conflict without feeling intimidated. A couple of people identified the need to take less control and let others have space to try things out. We discussed how we could express these PIGs in progressive, affirmative terms. For instance, 'being less controlling' was replaced with the more positive 'getting better at sharing control with others'.

We set up a system of accountability and support, with 'buddies' self-nominated across the team. We discussed our progress during Culture Club. We linked our learning to regular professional review and development cycles, adding heart back into a mandated workplace process that might easily lapse into cursory compliance.

Practising checking in every day, being upfront about values, having regular quarantined time to talk about how we were doing, and encouraging each other to consider where our personal growth intersected with being present at work – these things had a cumulative influence. People opened up, sharing their stories and placing their personal improvement goals in context. Collectively, we continued to change.

It sounds inspiring – but it wasn't easy. It was personally challenging. If I expected staff to get on board with bringing their whole selves to work, cultivating psychological safety, and growing personally, I would have to model this. At times I was courageous and modelled vulnerability. At other times I was self-protective. Sometimes, my efforts to be vulnerable went awkwardly wrong, and I found myself over sharing and emotionally bleeding on my colleagues – which didn't help anyone.

I aimed to improve managing the balance between courageous vulnerability and over sharing. I needed to achieve equanimity and be less reactive, to pause and think before I spoke. This was also important in receiving challenging feedback without becoming defensive.

One day, after a couple of complicated interactions that I had not handled well, one of my medical colleagues told me off.

'It felt pretty condescending – telling us things you know we already know,' she said.

I swallowed my pride and tendency to defend myself. I realised she was right. I apologised and thought about how to better manage this annoying know-it-all tendency.

❖❖❖

As we continued to work together, we grew as individuals and as a team. We started to see what the culture framework could look like in practice. Safety, growth and confidence resulted in stories of innovation and change from team members, some of whom had been rescued from the trauma of Oakden and others who had joined the team later.

I think, for instance, of Justin, an enrolled nurse with a background as a chef. Justin had worked at Oakden. Previously marginalised due to his eccentric loud-shirt-wearing quirkiness, Justin became as close to indispensable as it was possible to be. Besides being skilled in calmly delivering every aspect of personal care, he provided the in-house tech-guy expertise that every team needs. At an airport one day, Justin saw a 'magic motion box' projecting images that passers-by could interact with for a dynamic sensory experience. Full of enthusiasm, he rushed back, eager for us to become a technologically clever dementia care service, proposing we undertake a proof-of-concept project. He had already scoured the available technologies and started thinking about a pitch for funding.

Then I think of Bronnie, who had worked the night shift at Oakden, doing her best to deliver quality care but uninspired and undiscovered. It was Bronnie who had moved us all to tears with her reflective check-out during a Culture Club meeting, telling the story of her mother's life and death with dementia.

Bronnie was inspired to undertake the Bachelor of Dementia Care at the University of Tasmania, one of the world's best degrees of its type. She believed that her own life story meant she would struggle as a student. On the contrary, she excelled.

She became an influential, yet self-effacing, leader in our service. She intuitively understood what was happening for the person with dementia. She connected, engaged, and worked with people as if she was born to do it. She had an uncanny ability to sense what was troubling people, whether pain, anxiety or existential conflict. She would come in close alongside them, at their level, connecting with confident and warm physicality, speaking quietly and meaningfully. Because she *knew* their backstory, she knew how to help them. She did not see dementia, but rather the person, and she delighted in each one. I loved to hear her talk with family members.

'He's just such a lovely man,' she would say, with deep sincerity, of the resident she had managed to de-escalate from hitting another resident. She could pour oil on the most turbulent water.

As Bronnie grew in confidence and skill, we all learnt from her. But personal challenges come to everyone, often without warning. Bronnie began to feel tired and unwell. Following investigations, she was diagnosed with breast cancer. Her sudden disappearance from the team created an uncertain, troubled space. She was scheduled for surgery, and we all held out for good news.

After the operation, I received a text message from Bronnie: 'Thanks for all your kind thoughts,' she said. 'The surgery seems to have gone well, but I need to wait for my results. What's more important, though, is that they gave me this amazing single-use warm blanket – light as a feather and beautiful blue – but as warm as toast. I thought we could trial these with our people at Northgate House – it could be lovely and settling for them. I pinched mine so we can take a look!'

I couldn't help but laugh. My heart was warmed, as if I were wrapped up in a blanket myself, by Bronnie's selfless focus. Always thinking about how we could do better.

And then there was Michele, who had also come to Northgate House from Oakden, where he had worked as part of the original diversional therapy team. He was tall and tattooed, with long dark hair – a man whose appearance belied his gentle character. As an introvert, he would quietly go about his business, and it took many months before I could engage him in any exchange beyond a couple of awkwardly polite words. The trauma and turmoil of Oakden tossed Michele about in its wake. The mixed messages from the early staff forums, and the unions' strident influence, had resulted in Michele being unable to trust our efforts to have him move to Northgate House, despite the fact we were closing Oakden.

'No thank you,' he had said to me when asking him to move across, 'I don't want to work there. I'd rather stay here.'

But he was encouraged to give it a go, and, to his credit, he did.

Michele's reinvention was not instantaneous, but it was profound. He slowly built relationships with residents and team members and went from being a reticent outsider simply taking home a paycheque, to being a quiet achiever who went many extra miles. He was at the heart of the new team.

We had difficulty with some residents repeatedly pulling pictures off the wall, even when screwed on. We discovered that Michele could paint and commissioned him to cover some of the walls with colourful pictures that brought life to spaces where we could not hang a picture. At Christmas, Michele painted a full-size, flamboyantly festive Christmas tree on the wall in washable paint. Thanks to him, we all had a Christmas tree that posed no risk to our residents.

Supporting the team was Andrew, our occupational therapist. Andrew had worked competently for years in a generic community mental health job but had lost his gleam as an occupational therapist in his own right. He came to Northgate House with a need to redefine himself, and he did so brilliantly. His heart-of-gold, gregarious enthusiasm made him a reliable team builder, skilled in bringing people back together during times of dispute. In the spirit of the Culture Club, he developed a weekly meeting called 'Person of the Month' for any interested staff to brainstorm how we could provide better care for one of our most complex residents. At the end of the month, Andrew collated the findings and relayed the gems of understanding to the team. He invested in developing his sensory modulation knowledge as a therapy for people with dementia, believing that this would help him to help the rest of the team to work more skilfully. He was right.

This growth included learning to see everyone – team members and residents – generously and not write them off too quickly. Rob, another team member who had worked at Oakden, stretched upwards like a beanpole. He spoke bluntly, and, at first, I found myself cautious of him, but first impressions can be grossly misplaced. Like Bronnie, Rob demonstrated that he was a skilled, confident, calm and caring nurse, in contrast to his brusque exterior. He propelled others to be better.

One day I came upon Rob conversing with Dean, one of our residents who had developed vascular dementia after multiple strokes. Dean had been an intelligent and successful business owner, in charge of his domain. Following his illness, he had retained his energy and drive but lost his ability to communicate or understand the world around him. He had both receptive and expressive dysphasia – meaning that he could not understand what was said to him and could not find the words to match what he wanted to say. Full of thoughts he could not express, he could grow frustrated and irritable. Rob was skilled at turning the back-and-forth of apparently meaningless, out-of-context words into what looked like a satisfying interaction for both. Dean would make a statement, like tipping out a bowl of word salad. Rob would respond, connecting as best he could to the context, providing appropriate intonation and a genuine sense of interest, and turning a potentially agitating interaction into a satisfying one. It was adaptive and dignifying.

Barry, one of our much-loved residents, died following a rapid clinical deterioration. Barry's wife Gina had told Rob how much she loved a specific plant but had struggled to grow it herself. Rob brought in cuttings of the plant from his own garden as a gift for Gina.

'I hope she remembers us each time she sees this in her garden,' he said, misty-eyed, in our Culture Club debrief after Barry's death.

Jenie had joined our team as the carer consultant. She exemplified why it's essential to have people who have experience of caring for a family member themselves, working in all health and social care environments, with a focus on supporting people and their families from a carer's perspective. She was vivacious – a 'committed over sharer' in her own words. Before she came to us, she had no formal experience in this sort of work, having been a hospital sterilisation technician. Nevertheless, she brought deep knowledge from her time as the primary carer for her husband Kym, who had been diagnosed with dementia in his early forties. Over several years of rapid deterioration, Jenie and her family went through the best and the worst aspects of living with dementia. When she sat with families, she listened to them with the wisdom of having been there, and with her own intuitive gift of being able to offer comfort with just the right words. Jenie grew in leadership and in her determination to make a difference for people with younger-onset dementia. We had discovered a gem, and she had discovered a new career.

❖ ❖ ❖

One day, in the Culture Club, people started sharing stories of how they came to be working at Northgate House. Firstly, I was awestruck by the diversity of our team, people who came from different countries and cultures yet were able to gel with a shared commitment to our cause of compassionate care. Secondly, I was struck by the strength and determination they demonstrated, apparent in their remarkable tales of perseverance. It gave me a new appreciation of what personal growth might demand of us.

Many of our nursing team had travelled from other countries, enduring difficult transitions, roadblocks and painful sacrifices; but they had kept going, urged on by an aspiration to build different lives for their families and for themselves in Australia. Migration is typically highly stressful and can have a profound impact on mental health.[1] As I listened to my colleagues' stories, I marvelled at how they had triumphed over stressors and managed the practical, social, psychological and cultural challenges of navigating their way into Australian society and systems.

Surya was an outstanding nurse: calm, clever and caring. He was one of several Nepalese nurses who had joined our team. His gracious character and empathic ease were a gift to us. He carried himself with the quiet, humble confidence of an authentic leader, and it was no surprise to discover that he was a respected leader within his community. We rejoiced with Surya when his wife gave birth to their first child. We delighted in the celebrations of Deepawali, as our Nepalese colleagues effervesced with festivities in November. Our lives were enriched by diversity.

And yet, until Surya shared his story, I had been blissfully unaware of the poverty and unrelenting hard work he had endured to establish a life in Australia. There had been years spent living in meagre accommodation – a shed, a shack, shared rooms. While studying he had worked in multiple low-paid jobs, sending money home to his family. He'd had the most basic of diets. Year after year, digging deep, he held to a positive vision of the future. As he told his story, I gained a greater understanding of the power of delayed gratification and commitment to grow.

Norah had made her way to being a registered nurse at Northgate House via a complicated journey from Kenya. On first meeting her, it was easy to be mistaken into thinking she was a quiet, retiring person when, really, she was taking her time to assess the landscape and warm up. Once you got to know her, she revealed herself as dynamic, feisty and funny, ready to have a laugh and able to speak her mind with certainty.

Norah had left her children behind in Kenya, in the care of her mother and other family members, while she travelled ahead to secure their future in Australia. Everything was hard work across barriers of culture, communication and expectation. She encountered confusingly thick red tape as she navigated her nursing registration and managed her temporary visa. Each step of the pathway devoured time. Shortly after her children came to join her, she was confronted by the expiration of her visa and found herself in the Administrative Appeals Tribunal, pleading her case to remain in Australia. The Tribunal member presiding over her case – herself a devoted mother – listened to Norah's story and recognised the courage required to journey across the world to establish a new life for her children. After fearing the worst, at the eleventh hour, Norah was granted her visa to remain and continue building a secure future for her children, step by step.

Telling our stories

Gurmeet was gifted. He could support a person with dementia through the kind of personal care that could so easily be a source of distress, involving loss of dignity and a sense of exposure. Gurmeet's composure brought an infectious serene stillness, inspiring comfort and trust. Before coming to Australia, he had been a pharmacist and pharmaceutical sales representative in northern India. Despite coming on a skilled-worker visa, he had been unable to work as a pharmacist due to Australian registration processes, so he had retrained as an enrolled nurse, all the while maintaining life as a busy husband and father. While working at Northgate House, urged toward further growth, he decided to complete his registered nurse training, quickly progressing to graduation. We farewelled him in a bittersweet celebration, pleased that he would continue growing through new opportunities in the graduate nurse program.

Febin felt a vocational calling to become a nurse, just before he finished training as a dentist, also in India. He weathered parental disappointment at his career change, redeeming himself only through his decision to relocate his young family to Australia, which was considered to carry a level of prestige. By the time he joined our team as nurse unit manager, Febin had developed adeptness in management and leadership through some tough gigs in residential aged care. He was informed by strong moral principles and a devotion to putting others first. He embraced every new demand with grace. I was challenged by his constant desire to do better as he sought honest feedback from all team members – listening, learning, and writing notes to himself about his personal improvement goals. He pinned these goals at his eye-line above his desk, to be reminded daily of his commitment to grow.

Then there was Bindu, who joined the team as our nurse consultant. In the Culture Club, Bindu told a story about being newly married in India. With great expectation, her husband had travelled to Kuwait for a job that turned out to be too good to be true. He found himself caught up in a dangerous industrial scam, and Bindu was left scraping together every last saving the young couple had to get him home.

Through dogged persistence, Bindu and her family eventually made their way to the UK and then Australia. What was most striking about Bindu was her determination to grow and be a better version of herself, not just as a well-studied and skilful nurse, but as a person. 'I know I can be rigid and reactionary,' she acknowledged with vulnerability, 'but I tell things as I see them – and I'm learning and changing.' She was right, and the team came to love her for it.

Andrew and Anthony, the Truong brothers – occupational therapist and physiotherapist, respectively – shared their experience of being born in Australia to Chinese–Vietnamese parents. Their parents had escaped from war-decimated Vietnam to Thailand and on to Australia on an overcrowded boat, experiencing profound trauma that they would not even speak of. They gave their two boys anglicised names hoping that it would make their lives in Australia more straightforward. We were all moved as we considered the price that Andrew and Anthony's parents had paid for the promise of a more hopeful life for their sons.

Safwat, our clinical pharmacist, started by explaining: 'Identity has always been a challenge for me. It's been hard to know where I belong.' His parents were Egyptian Coptic Christians living in Sudan. They had separated, and Safwat's mother had moved with Safwat – a young child – to the UK before eventually migrating to Australia. He flourished in his studies and became an outstanding pharmacist but with a lingering unsettledness from a life of multiple transitions. I gained a deep respect for Safwat, as I did for all my other colleagues, as I listened to their stories. It was humbling, working with remarkable people.

Many others joined our team and took to our developing way of working, sharing themselves and their stories. Dan, the broad-shouldered podiatrist with a walrus moustache, was always amiable and never frightened despite the possibility that, should he put a foot wrong, he might get a kick in the teeth. Being skilled in reading residents' moods, it never happened. Emma, our receptionist, young and growing into the workplace's challenges, struggled at home with her father's diagnosis of motor neurone disease. When met with kindness and given opportunity, Emma blossomed; she would pitch in and get things done. Many nurses joined the team, drawn by the promise of a supportive workplace but then contributing to its development themselves – all in the face of the continual demands of working at the most physically demanding end of dementia care.

❖❖❖

What also happened, as we encouraged each other to be better, was that people gained confidence to solve problems and innovate. Solutions had to be simple and low-cost – but we had some fun moments as we created ways around the challenges of daily life in delivering care.

We had a recurrent problem with some of the men who lived in our care pressing the bright red fire alarm button. They were drawn to it like a beacon. Regulations meant that we could not move it somewhere less accessible. It was an expensive problem, with bills mounting into several thousand dollars for repeated needless visits from the fire service. Thinking about the changes in visual perception in people with dementia, Antonietta, our nurse unit manager at the time, proposed we stick a pattern of bright red dots of various sizes around the fire alarm as a visual distraction and see what happens. The experiment was a success. We never had another inappropriate pressing of the fire alarm.

Another problem resulting from the changed visual perception of the men we provided care for was their tendency to walk into walls, corners and door frames. This underpins the dementia design principle that calls for clear cues and visual contrasts to help people with dementia find their way. Because our renovation had occurred in great haste during a crisis, inadequate attention had been paid to this issue. One day I arrived at Northgate House to find that Bronnie, Andrew and Michele had slopped some brightly coloured paint on all the doorframes and corners encountered by our residents. 'Don't worry, it'll wash off with water,' Bronnie reassured. It looked a bit messy, but it worked a treat. We had no more awkward collisions.

There was a time when a problem like this would have been accepted as something we had to tolerate. Later on, we were able to repaint properly, which looked much better.

Anthony, our physiotherapist, worked all sorts of angles to get permission to access the hydrotherapy pool at a nearby hospital. There were challenges in managing issues like continence and cleaning, but he set up a remarkable program for people with advanced dementia, supported enthusiastically by Michele, Justin and Andrew. We discovered that our resident Kathy could throw a water polo ball through a hoop. On her first visit to the pool, Sally, who had not been in the water for years, instinctively lay back and floated, completely relaxed – a far cry from the agitation she sometimes experienced. This was the outcome of our team being given a safe space to have a go at things, of recognising that not everything will work, and of being constantly encouraged to find better ways of being and doing.

Of course, people sometimes moved on from our team. Some retired. Some decided that the work was not for them. Others decided our *way* of working was not for them. We learnt to go with the flow – to not see these people as a problem that created more system gaps, but to consider their departures as a sign that they were moving towards clarification of their values and determining what personal growth looked like for them. Having picked up the infectious growth orientation, others moved on to opportunities that would compel further growth. Departures could be difficult; we were saying goodbye to friends, often tearfully facing the challenge of recruiting new people with like values. I took to reminding the team that no one stays anywhere forever. What was important was that people had the opportunity to flourish.

❖ ❖ ❖

Throughout this process, we had genuine senior leadership support, championed by our CEO, who gave us the go-ahead to experiment and learn – having a go at something counter-cultural. Everything about our project demonstrated the benefit of bottom-up, not top-down, change. It was crucial to give those who delivered daily services and care a sense of empowerment and ownership. Deliberate steps to democratise the workforce created an environment in which people could 'buy in' to the way we wanted to work. From recruitment to everyday behaviour, we talked about our values and sincerely sought to put them into practice. We didn't get everything right. Missteps and mistakes continued to present themselves like reliable tutors. We made space for innovations, some of which were triumphant. In a microcosmic melting pot, with cultures, conflicts, stories and experiences continually unfolding around us, the alignment of leadership and support enabled growth and change.

Andrew and the Uncharted Leadership team provided us with skilled facilitation, which helped us co-create a meaningful way of working. They were active, curious and flexible. They coached and mentored, and as we became more confident and capable, they gradually withdrew and left us to it. After completing their work with us, they moved on to use the insights they gained from our project to contribute constructive change in other organisations. Culture change requires investment – there is an outlay of time, effort and resources, but the dividends far exceed the costs. What we learnt, and the Uncharted Leadership team demonstrated in other settings after leaving us, is that change is achievable with sincere intentionality, modest investment, and committed persistence. The importance of this work is not just for the severe cases, like ours, in need of significant remediation – it is transportable and adds value to any team. I advocate that the lessons described here are relevant to all other health and social care settings. There is no reason why this type of transformative work cannot be employed everywhere. That's the universal – *everyone* – relevance of this story.

❖ ❖ ❖

We came through a second accreditation with commendations. We underwent announced and unannounced inspections from the Office of the Chief Psychiatrist and the Community Visitor's Scheme, even at

9 pm on a Friday night, when least expected. We had an independent evaluation of the outcomes of our residents who had previously lived at Oakden. We remained a work in progress, with each external assessment providing evidence of transformation. Nurses know nurses, so we had no trouble recruiting. People wanted to join our team because, although the work was hard, the support was rich.

During evaluation of our growth culture project, team members were interviewed about their experiences. The dominant theme reflected the humanising of our workforce.

'Now we start with kindness and generosity,' said one team member.

'I feel physically and mentally better,' said another.

'You remember why you fell in love with the job,' said yet another.

One team member captured the flow-on impact of investment in our people. 'Happier staff,' they summarised, 'means happier residents and happier families.'

The consequence of transforming culture and morale was transformed care for the people we served.[2]

The impact of all this learning, changing and growing was captured most eloquently by Nicola, from our cleaning and catering team. After a robust discussion in the Culture Club, she paused when it came to her turn to check out. She quietly declared: 'I like what we're becoming.'

The wisdom and vision of her words remain with me, a reminder of the dynamic, vital nature of our working and living. We are not a final product or a static endpoint. We are 'becoming', and our task is to find a way to stay openhearted, learning and giving along the way.

17

Trauma and transformation

Listening to each other's stories – discovering our distinctiveness, while finding common ground – brought about change. And as our culture changed, the way we delivered care changed, emerging as we turned our attention to the stories of the people in our care.

After opening Northgate House, we commenced the Life Story Project, led by Jane, our first carer consultant. The project involved developing a rich personal biography of every person in our care. It was not a new strategy; many quality providers of health and aged care have placed a priority on activities like this and the evidence is that knowing a person's story can change how the person is seen and how care is delivered.[1] Even quick-to-use tools, such as the 'Top Five', used in many hospitals to list essential personal information from the person's or carer's perspective, represent a step in the right direction, reminding everyone involved that the person receiving care is precisely that – a person.[2]

In our project, stories, photos, anecdotes and personal preferences were gathered and drafted into a first-person account of each person's life. With the families' collaboration and approval, these were printed and displayed in the person's room, where families could enjoy them, and staff could absorb them. The stories were translated into care plans and clinical discussions, guiding our understanding, and making the *person* a priority over their illness.

AN EVERYONE STORY

The life-story project triggered a cascade of discovery. The very first story we documented belonged to a woman called Maisie. Her story, in this context, is all about how we changed because of what she taught us.

❖❖❖

When I first met Maisie, she was sitting in a chair at the end of a corridor in Oakden. She was a small woman who had the air of a wildling, with dishevelled salt-and-pepper hair, mismatched clothing and the dried remnants of an earlier meal patterning her front. She appeared agitated and hypervigilant, ready to protect her corner from any wandering co-resident or passing staff member.

Maisie was another one of our residents who had receptive and expressive dysphasia – difficulty understanding what was said to her and communicating her thoughts and needs. She managed to utter jumbled phrases, dominated by repetitive syllables and punctuated at times by swear words, which she spat out like bullets. It's a curious thing that, for many people, the part of the brain that enables us to swear is one of the last regions of the speech centre to succumb to Alzheimer's disease. This partly explains why some people who had never previously uttered a curse begin swearing like a trooper when living with Alzheimer's disease.

Maisie's family were deeply troubled. Ever since her diagnosis with younger-onset dementia, life had been tough. Initially she had been able to cope at home, but as her illness progressed, she needed to go into residential aged care. She presented with high levels of anxiety and then behaviours that limited the delivery of care. Eventually, her first facility decided that they could not provide Maisie with the care she needed. She went to the local general hospital, where she had medication changes and, with higher levels of staff, she settled a little. She was then transferred to a new facility, and a short while later the same problems re-emerged, only worse. This went on several times until, during one hospital admission to an older persons' mental health unit when things were not settling, the doctors advised the family that Maisie needed to be referred to Oakden. There was nowhere else to go.

The tumult of travelling back and forth between the hospital and aged care was distressing. The family were relieved that this cycle would now stop, but they also felt deep guilt for placing Maisie at Oakden.

At Oakden, Maisie was regarded as aggressive and hostile. At times the staff would respond by ignoring her, leaving her to sit alone and unattended. Providing support for personal care and hygiene was particularly difficult. Maisie would become hysterical during bathing and toileting routines – screaming, hitting, spitting and biting. It was horrible for her and the staff. At Oakden, four or sometimes five staff would hold her firmly to remove her clothing, bathe her, and manage her continence.

Maisie was among the first residents to move from Oakden to Northgate House. Viewed simply from the perspective of her characteristic behaviours, it would have been easy to describe her as 'difficult', 'combative', 'resistant' and even 'dangerous'. Still, we knew that looking at her through this lens was not okay. As we delved into Maise's story, we got beyond the behaviours that grabbed attention so easily. We started to understand the 'why' of her responses and got to know a rich and complex person.

❖ ❖ ❖

Maisie was born in a small market town in the UK during the Second World War. She was born ten minutes after her twin brother, Stephen, and the two remained close throughout their lives. Maisie's father was in the merchant navy and, when war came, he joined the Royal Navy. The war brought Maisie's father to Australia, to help defend against the advancing Japanese forces. After the war, Maisie's father disembarked in Sydney and remained there.

In 1946, Maisie's mother brought the children to Australia to reunite the family as 'ten-pound Poms' – part of a scheme that resulted in a large migration from the UK in the years after the war. The family lived in western Sydney for a couple of years but then moved to South Australia. They lived in Adelaide before settling in the remote coastal fishing town of Port Lincoln.

Maisie was a good student at school and grew into a beautiful young woman. Many years later, she still looked back at winning the Miss Port Lincoln Beauty Contest at seventeen as one of her life's highlights. She married for the first time a short while later – before she had turned eighteen – and gave birth to three children before she was twenty-one.

Life could be difficult as a young mother in remote rural South Australia in the 1960s. Ominous themes that wended through Maisie's life began to affect her mental health. The darkest secret – her father's sexual abuse – left deep wounds that revisited her in unexpected ways. She experienced violence from her first husband. Seeking to dull the pain of the trauma, Maisie drank. She fought back at her husband, and the violence spilled onto her children. This later became the greatest regret of her life, as she reflected on the broken relationships with her children.

Divorce led to a second marriage, where similar patterns of violence were repeated. And so, to a third marriage, where, for a time, things settled. Life reached a hiatus of happiness, travel and peace. But in 2006, when Maisie was in her early sixties, she and her husband were in a car accident. A vehicle slammed into the side of their car, with Maisie in the passenger's side, and pinned it against a tree. The car burst into flames and Maisie survived by being dragged through the vehicle's rear, just in time.

For the next four years, Maisie was ensnared in an agonising struggle with post-traumatic stress disorder. She repeatedly relived her near-death experience and continuously tried to numb the anxiety. This took its toll.

In 2010, as her father lay dying in hospital, Maisie wrestled with unresolved trauma. At this point, her third husband decided it was time to end the marriage. Her children remained distant. Except for her twin brother, Maisie's faithful friend through the years, she was alone.

Then, a little more than a year later, following worsening problems with her memory, confusion, and ability to cope with life, Maisie was diagnosed with dementia. It seems impossible to make sense of some stories. Why do some people appear to live charmed lives while others experience a devastating burden of trauma and loss?

As we probed into Maisie's story, not only did we begin to appreciate the impact of trauma on her life, but we also discovered a complex, creative and captivating woman. Despite areas of instability in her personal life, she had held the same job as an administrative assistant for close to forty years. She had loved her work and was valued in her workplace. She maintained a Christian faith throughout her life, albeit not always in the institutional church. We learnt of her fondness for gardens and her delight in flowers. She loved to read, watch movies, and she had an enduring passion for the music of the sixties and seventies. We learnt that she had been meticulously concerned about fashion and grooming, from before she won the beauty pageant at seventeen. She'd always loved a trip to the hairdresser. Maisie's brother provided pictures of an immaculate and beautiful woman – in stark contrast to the dishevelled person I first met onsite at Oakden.

Maisie provided the staff at Northgate House, individually and as a community, with an epiphany. Our task was to understand and honour her story as we cared for her. We celebrated the joyful gemstones we unearthed in her history. We also came to understand how trauma had impacted her experiences and relationships, and how these emerged in the context of dementia and receiving care.

The turning point came when the staff realised the extent to which the delivery of care compelled Maisie to revisit her earlier trauma experiences. They realised that Maisie was not the problem. She was not being 'difficult' or 'combative'. What we were doing to her was the problem. Every time the staff removed her clothes, she felt exposed. The memory of trauma is held in the body, without conscious awareness.[3] In simply going to the bathroom, Maisie's trauma-sensitive fight-or-flight mechanism, driven by her brain's deep emotion centres, fired off. With that came Maisie's efforts to protect herself – to remain safe.

A couple of the nurses experimented. They changed the way they supported Maisie through bathing. Recognising that Maisie felt threatened by crowded and noisy environments, a deliberate choice was made to limit the number of staff in the room to two people. Maisie was never left fully unclothed or exposed. The nurses wrapped her in soft towels to keep her warm and covered. Maisie's favourite music was played quietly in the background, and aromatherapy was used to further soften and sweeten the atmosphere. One of the nurses would get down to Maisie's level, make eye contact, hold her hand gently and talk to her consistently, explaining what they were doing in a quiet voice and straightforward language. The delivery of care – and, in turn, Maisie's experience – completely turned around.

The behaviours that had been so problematic quickly resolved. Everything was different. Maisie's mealtimes became more relaxed, and she healthily gained weight. Personal hygiene care became a time of warmth and sensory comfort for her. There was no more defensiveness or anxiety. Only one staff member was needed to work with Maisie for bathing. She started enjoying visits from the hairdresser. Her brother brought new clothes in for her. In direct contrast to my first encounter with her, I arrived at Northgate House one day to find Maisie sitting in a comfy chair in the sun, dressed beautifully and with a stylish new haircut.

Maisie spent time in the garden. She delighted in outings on the community bus, holding hands with one of the nurses. She would try hard to communicate, searching for words to connect with the people who had become like a family to her. Her favourite pastime was to sit in a lounge chair and hum along to the movie *Mamma Mia!*, which took her back to the beloved Abba songs that had defined the 1970s for her.[4] (We all listened to that movie *way* too many times.) Her most beautiful moments were when she was sitting quietly, hand in hand with her twin brother, the two of them not needing to talk but just able to *be*.

Maisie was sincerely loved by the staff at Northgate House. Somewhere, through deeply learning her story, she stopped being someone with dementia. She was Maisie. A person with a life tapestry coloured by highs and lows, and with trauma that needed to be understood with compassion.

Maisie's brother, Stephen, captured what the paradigm shift meant for him in a simple letter of thanks:

Heartfelt thanks to all the staff at Northgate House for the care and support given to my twin sister since she moved there from Oakden. She is now rarely distressed. She's never aggressive and is so much calmer and happier. Everyone is so caring and friendly. They take time to talk with us and do whatever is needed to make sure Maisie is comfortable.

I'm sure it's their care and attention that has made it more like a home than an institution. I cannot speak too highly of the work everyone does. I know that Maisie is as precious to the staff as she is to me.

Eventually, Maisie no longer needed to be in a specialist service like Northgate House. Working with her brother, we organised her transition to a good-quality residential aged care home. There were tears as she left, and an especially pedantic handover to her new home from the team, anxious that those taking over Maisie's care should not lose sight of her story.

18

It all comes together

Learning requires multiple inputs to become embedded. Our team witnessed the outcome of listening carefully to each person's story, as we had with Maisie, allowing it to inform how we served them. This success watered the seeds of creative care, which were joyously championed within the team. They had made the connection between stories, culture and care, and recognised the benefits.

We accepted a referral for David, a sixty-three-year-old man with younger-onset dementia. He had been through a terrible time. The facility he'd been living in could not cope with his outbursts of extreme aggression, and he spent months in hospital. At times he appeared settled and would even sit and look at, if not read, the newspaper and have semi-coherent conversations. At other times he would be distressed and agitated. He maintained his strength, and when perturbed, he could inflict significant damage on anyone or anything in his way. As was so often the case, times of personal care were a problem. At worst, he had seven care staff in the hospital, holding him to manage his hygiene care. At other times, when stressed, he would break furniture and terrify those nearby. During his time in hospital, the staff had initiated numerous 'code blacks' where security officers had been called to restrain him. His unpredictability and extreme behaviours were so significant that there seemed no alternative but to treat him with multiple psychotropic medications in high doses. Everyone was on high alert, including David.

It all comes together

In assessing his referral, our nurse unit manager, Antonietta, visited David in the hospital. She read everything she could about him and discovered he was a veteran who'd been in the navy. Antonietta gleaned from the team looking after him that he appeared more suspicious when surrounded by men in uniforms. She brought that information to our interdisciplinary team to discuss how we might best help David. We agreed that he needed to come to Northgate House and prepared for his transfer.

Suspecting that the uniforms might trigger David's anxiety, Justin suggested the team wear casual clothes when David arrived and while he settled in. We wanted him to feel at home, and everyone agreed. In some services, staff always wear regular street clothes, but at Northgate House, the team usually wore nursing uniforms. When he arrived, they were wearing coloured T-shirts or casual clothes.

David did settle, but not without episodes of agitation. Jenie, our carer consultant, worked with his son to collect a rich life story, and his behaviour began to make more sense. As a young man, David had joined the navy but did not see active service. In his first week, he experienced bullying from senior colleagues; this culminated in David falling down a ladder – the height of a full deck – and crushing both ankles. The event became a defining one for him, spawning a slow rehabilitation, chronic pain and residual post-traumatic stress disorder that revisited him for years.

This story gave us a better understanding of the issues that emerged through David's anxious and defensive behaviours in dementia. We recognised that he was sensitive to noise and crowding; his agitation increased when other people – particularly men – came into his space. We tracked the pattern of his chronic pain and were better able to provide him with pain relief as a preference over other medications.

We also learnt that David had a cheeky sense of humour. He would march around the unit arm in arm with Bronnie, laughing at the slightest burp or sneeze. We also learnt that David liked to be protective of our female staff. If he perceived that one of them was in a situation of risk, he would rally to their defence. This required the team to be on the lookout, ready to step in and redirect David or those around him when the pressure cooker environment built up steam.

❖❖❖

The significance of trauma as an influencing factor for many of our residents was demonstrated over and over. There are some cases where behavioural and psychological symptoms of dementia occur as neuropsychiatric sequelae of the illness, and not necessarily as indicators of an unmet need or underlying vulnerability. Nevertheless, we observed a clear pattern between traumatic histories and the emergence of distressing symptoms.

The experience of trauma is widespread and effects people in diverse ways.[1] The impact of trauma can be immediate or delayed. It can be severe and acute, or more subtle and chronic. Trauma can impact long-term psychological and physical health outcomes.[2]

Anyone in a healthcare system, whether receiving care or providing it, may have experienced trauma. This may profoundly impact on their interactions within that system. *Trauma-informed care* is an important approach, relevant to all health and social care systems (to every system, actually) that understand this and seek to avoid retraumatising people, or causing new trauma.[3]

I raise it here, not to provide another term of healthcare jargon to confuse you, but because taking a trauma-informed approach is such an important part of us finding a kinder, more effective and empowering way to work with *all* people. In this way, *trauma-informed care* is closely aligned with *person-centred care*. In practice, this means shifting perspective; rather than asking, 'What's wrong with you?' ask the more curious, 'What happened to you?' This offers the hope of, 'How can I help you?'[4]

At Northgate House, our care was transformed as we recognised this important relationship between trauma and people's interactions, and how we could either make things worse – or better – simply by understanding the person's experience.

It all comes together

❖❖❖

Anybody who met George, a man in his eighties with a tussled head of grey hair and a slight stoop, could tell he was intelligent. He seemed sophisticated and cultured. Dementia had not entirely taken words from him and, in the most subdued of voices, he would try and communicate, lapsing between his various languages: English, Croatian and Italian. It was necessary to listen very carefully to catch snatches of meaning before he became irritated by his listener's failure to understand.

George's daughter filled his room with his favourite things. Pictures and books revealed his love of European culture and history – art, food, music, architecture. As we got to know him, we discovered a complex and perplexing story that helped us understand him as he lived with dementia.

Olga, our nurse who spoke Croatian, listened carefully to George, hearing a story of torrid trauma, of being interned in a concentration camp and struggling to survive. He told of having witnessed his father's murder during the war. This history of trauma was not unknown; he had described it many times over the years, and it was recorded in the clinical history handed to us by previous care providers. It made some sense of his rapid escalations in anxiety, followed by behaviour that appeared to be self-protective, but which was potentially dangerous.

We sought to better understand George's story. But then, during a meeting with our team one day, his daughter dropped a bombshell.

'I'm sorry to rain on the parade,' she said, 'but his story of trauma – about his father's death – it's not true.'

There were several of us sitting around the table, and our jaws dropped. His account had appeared so convincing, and so many care providers had documented the same details before us. As I reflected on the story's elements, I recognised inconsistencies – but I still perceived real trauma underpinning George's distress and behaviour.

'Dad didn't see his father murdered,' George's daughter told us. 'His father left him. He walked out on his wife and my dad – abandoned them when my dad was six years old.'

A different story of trauma began to emerge.

'His father was killed,' she went on, 'but my dad didn't see it. His mother received a letter telling her about it sometime later. He wasn't in a concentration camp, although he knew people who were.'

George's daughter, a clinical psychologist, provided her understanding of what had happened to George.

'He was very damaged by his father's abandonment and created an alternative account that managed the pain and insult of that loss. It was viewed with greater sympathy than the truth. His distress resulted in him struggling to manage his emotions and behaviour – leading to an impulsive temper. As a young man, he fled Croatia after threatening his mother with a knife and being wanted by the police. He eventually made his way to Australia and spent the rest of his life telling grandiose stories that compensated for that early loss and its impact – the story of his father's murder was the pinnacle of all those stories.'

The revelation from his daughter regarding the truth of George's trauma – and how it had shaped his character, life and relationships – begged the question of how this carefully cultivated narrative had come to be handed over between different care teams as accepted fact. Our team reflected on the need to embrace people's stories without losing our sense of inquisitiveness, and to work to deeper understand people's experiences. The revelation also challenged us to talk more enquiringly with families and carers to confirm and explore the meaning of stories. We realised how easy it is for care teams to miss important interactions with family members when focused on the immediate concerns of day-to-day care. They don't necessarily open up if we don't provide the time and space – and actually ask them.

We might have judged George for such elaborate deception. But it was essential to counterbalance this disturbing revelation with the evident warmth that his daughter maintained for him – tempered by a realistic appraisal of his faults.

It all comes together

'It became his truth,' she said to us, 'because the actual truth was too confronting for him. He could not reconcile the thought that his father did not love him enough to stay. That's the real trauma.'

Throughout his life, George had lost himself in work. His marriage had failed, but he maintained a connection with his daughter – albeit from a distance. For twenty-five years, before becoming unwell with dementia, he had lived alone on a property of multiple acres, oscillating between trips away to Europe for work and culture, and immersing himself in the development of an expansive, meticulous garden. His intelligence and high level of functioning offered compensation but did not resolve his internal conflict.

'I don't remember him ever stopping moving – even when he sat down, he seemed agitated,' his daughter told us. 'And he kept himself protected, away from people. I can only imagine it must be difficult for him now, having to live so close to others and rely on staff for help.'

The complex trauma of George's lost relationship with his father, and its impact on his identity, informed our development of his care plan. We were alert to his agitation and remembered the potential for explosions of temper – just like when he had accosted his mother many decades earlier. One day, the staff deftly intercepted him picking up a rock he'd dug up in the garden to use as a defensive weapon after his temper had been triggered.

We carefully supported the sanctity of his personal space and belongings, knowing that incursions could prompt defensiveness against perceived exposure. We respected his need for deference – to be treated as an important person. We came to understand and enjoy George, seeing someone who had managed to make his way through a life of challenges, wounds and opportunities as best he could.

❖ ❖ ❖

Another of our residents at Northgate House, Rosalyn – a seventy-two-year-old woman from one of South Australia's beautiful vineyard regions – shared similarities with George but had her own story. Diagnosed with frontotemporal dementia, in some ways, she had less disability than many of our residents. She could hold a superficially sensible conversation – provided her listener could roll with the lapses in social appropriateness typical of someone with this type of dementia. She retained the ability to manage parts of her personal care, with a nurse standing by to prompt her. She enjoyed picking flowers but, because of her inability to moderate this activity, would eagerly strip the garden of every breakable branch and stem to present her momentary favourite team member with a bouquet. Our garden at Northgate House took a beating for a while.

So why was Rosalyn in a specialist service for people with extreme symptoms? She was fiercely defensive of the physical environment she believed belonged to her, and her borders extended well beyond her room. She retained exceptional hearing, and the opening of the door from the garden by a passing nurse or resident would trigger Rosalyn's eruption from her room. She was quick and decisive, and the passer-by could be set upon with ferocity. While we worked through strategies to understand and help moderate Rosalyn's behaviour, there were repeated incidents – fortunately without serious injury, but with much alarm. There was no way that a mainstream aged care home could manage such extreme behaviour, so she had come to live in our care.

Rosalyn's continual anxiety and vigilance made more sense after a meeting with her family, who told us her story. Rosalyn always maintained that she'd had a happy marriage, but the truth was very different. Her husband had been unpredictable. Likely depressed, he had spent many hours in the shed, drinking alone. Rosalyn spent nights awake, remaining on guard to protect her children from her husband's temper when he eventually re-entered the house. Rosalyn's children were unsure of how much their father had physically harmed Rosalyn, but they were confident she had lived in constant fear and psychological distress – always on alert. Despite this, she had remained a warm and much-loved member of her community in country South Australia, faithful to her local church, kind and busy. We saw both sides of Rosalyn, and better understood the themes of defence and protection.

It all comes together

❖❖❖

It wasn't only the uncovering of these stories of trauma that changed the way we worked. Discovering what made our residents tick, in an environment dedicated to compassionate care, with permission to learn and grow, also contributed significantly.

Gigi was one of our first residents at Northgate House, having moved from Oakden with us. She was in her late seventies and living with Alzheimer's disease. At Oakden, she had been mainly confined to a princess chair, reclined to the point that she could not get up, held in place with a lap restraint belt. Like many of our residents, Gigi had lost most of her language, but she would call out loudly in distress. She would writhe her legs and bite her hand. She would grab her knee, pulling it up toward her mouth as she called out, or rub at it repeatedly until it became calloused. It doesn't take long for the human body to become deconditioned in a princess chair, and when she arrived at Northgate House, Gigi could not walk.

There was much to consider in improving her situation. We all know that too much time lying down, not moving, results in discomfort. Gigi spent all her time restricted in the same position. There was no doubt that pain was a central issue for her. We explored Gigi's story and realised how much being active had meant to her. She'd been an athlete from childhood and throughout her adult years. She'd been a champion golfer, out on the golf course several times each week in retirement, able to swing the five iron and belt the ball far down the fairway. It was obvious: Gigi needed to move. And yet she was strapped in a chair, immobilised and in pain.

Within days of Gigi arriving at Northgate House, Anthony, our physiotherapist, had her upright – him on one side and a nurse on the other. Within weeks she was walking again, at first with support and then a few steps by herself. She would tire and need to sit, and we ordered her a new chair, measured to fit her correctly. There were no restraints on site, and she was never tied down again. Her daily routine was developed around the regular times she was helped to stand and assisted to walk around the unit and garden. Still living with dementia, Gigi continued to have episodes of agitation, but her life was now very different. We continued to manage her pain, using a combination of medication, massage and regular movement. Her appetite improved. She gained weight, just as Maisie had done.

Gigi's husband, Bruce, was transformed by the relief of seeing this improvement. Bruce visited every day except Wednesday – his golfing day – and became a part of the Northgate House family. There was a particularly special moment when the team surprised Bruce and Gigi with a beautifully set table, with sparkling wine, flowers and celebratory cake for their fiftieth wedding anniversary. Bruce was so well known that an astute catering staff member noticed him one day sitting beside Gigi with one side of his face drooping. She raised the alarm, and Bruce was rushed to hospital. He'd had a stroke, which was caught at the very earliest moments, possibly saving his life, and certainly saving him from disability. It all comes together.

Then there was Gerard, a short-statured man in his seventies with a jovial disposition that emerged between episodes of distress and agitation. Before coming to us, he had caused great consternation in his aged care home and the hospital, with staff often finding him crawling on the floor, looking like he was plucking things from the wall. Had he fallen? Why was he doing that?

His care providers did not feel able to allow Gerard to self-manage this behaviour. He needed help to get up and be distracted, but a short while later would be found attending to some invisible issue beneath the handrail again. When he arrived at Northgate House, the team encountered the same issues.

We learnt that Gerard had been a vigneron. He had owned a vineyard and made wines that sold well. He had spent a lifetime low to the ground, pruning, tying up and harvesting from his beloved vines. His behaviour made more sense. We discovered Gerard was quite capable of getting up from his kneeling position when he was ready. By looking at his behaviour through the lens of his story, we became less anxious and more tolerant. We focused on how we could use this knowledge to provide more satisfying opportunities for him to reconnect with a meaningful activity: we gave him grapes to pick and plants to dig into the garden.

We were less perplexed when, sometime later, a new resident, Marcus, started doing a similar thing – he would get down on the floor and appear to be measuring and lining things up. 'Don't worry about that,' said his wife calmly, 'he spent his life laying tiles.'

Another resident, Dino, insisted on scrubbing his hands and arms up to his elbows. It made sense when we considered his years working as a mechanic, always cleaning off sticky black grease. He appeared grounded by the practice – so the team simply went with it.

But 'Nug' was an enigma. Like so many of the people we cared for, he had lost his ability to talk, so couldn't tell us his story – but when he was happy, he would light up with the broadest, toothiest laugh. He was a stocky man in his late sixties and had no family that we could find. His guardians – the rotating, overworked social workers from the Office of the Public Advocate – had minimal personal information about him. This hampered their ability to make decisions on his behalf, as much as it posed challenges for us in understanding how best to care for him. We managed to trace his history to a tiny, remote country town in the South Australian outback, where we discovered he'd been a regular at the pub. It seemed that Nug's life had centred around a straightforward routine. He drove trucks – they were his passion. This glimpse into his world gave us the key to easing his episodes of agitation.

Nug loved to travel with other residents on a minibus, on trips from the beach to the hills. He insisted on sitting in the front passenger's seat, or right behind the driver, where he could see the road disappearing under the bonnet, while being swayed by the vehicle's repetitive movement, evoking the body-held, wordless memory of his years behind the wheel, rumbling along the vast, flat expanses of South Australian transit routes. The only difficulty was when it came time to get off the bus. It was his favourite place to be.

❖❖❖

As we got to know the people in our care, we took a keen interest in details such as their musical tastes. There is much evidence supporting the therapeutic value of music for people with dementia.[5] The research shows that targeting music to the person's history and personal tastes will enhance the therapeutic benefit.[6, 7] I'm reminded of the distinctive choices of three of our residents who all lived along the same corridor. For each, music was a vital ingredient in their care plan, creating meaning and connection with their earlier lives, and soothing them at times of distress. We supplied each with a set of headphones and a customised playlist, developed with their families.

Barry, who was in his mid-seventies, had been diagnosed with progressive supranuclear palsy, an illness that had not only caused dementia but changed his gait and gaze, resulting in a glazed expression and persistent falls, usually straight backwards. He had a cheeky sense of humour, which he retained until very late in his illness. He also maintained his passion for jazz, with broad tastes from the Great American Songbook to more avant-garde artists. The music eased his moments of agitation and provided him with a rich source of pleasure.

A couple of doors down the hallway lived Philippe, a Frenchman, just turned seventy, slender and strong from years of regular attendance at the gym. His wife was a retired anaesthetist who thoroughly understood the clinical aspects of Philippe's care. She visited most days and continued to find the daily realities of living with dementia distressing. The illness had left Philippe without language and caused reflexive, defensive behaviour and extremely loud vocalisation. Despite this, Philippe carried an air of European sophistication. He had a long-standing love of classical music and the arts. Noise, excess activity, and pop music agitated him. Quiet time in his room listening to Chopin's nocturnes, or Debussy, or Schubert's lieder, provided solace and comfort.

In contrast to Philippe, Doug carried himself like a larrikin. He was sixty-nine and had come to Northgate House several years after his diagnosis with younger-onset dementia. Like Nug, he had driven trucks for a living – and a passion – and had spent years driving long-haul trips through the night. Not surprisingly, sleeping at night was one of Doug's biggest challenges. It was unrealistic of us to expect that he would simply adopt a normal daily rhythm, given that he had not lived that way during his adult life. He was incredibly tall – around two metres – so lying in bed was also problematic. The trouble was that Doug didn't sleep during the day, either. He had arrived at Northgate House from a hospital where he'd wandered the ward incessantly, climbing over furniture and falling over, which was frightening given how far it was to the ground.

Doug also loved music and had a particular favourite – Queen. We discovered that Freddie Mercury's soaring vocals held Doug's attention so he could sit and rest for a while. By reflecting on his story, changing our expectations, and not forcing him into a routine that suited us rather than him, and by exploring how his long-held preferences could help us help him – along with some carefully prescribed medication – his sleeping improved. He became less agitated and fell over less frequently.

❖❖❖

There was one resident of Northgate House whose illness bewildered us more than anyone else's. Kathy lived with the rare form of genetically conferred, younger-onset, frontotemporal dementia, caused by the C9orf72 gene that can also cause motor neurone disease. On one level, she was profoundly disabled, yet she retained remarkable skills. It was as if Kathy's form of dementia functioned like an acquired autism, locking her away from being able to express herself. Most of the time, she had minimal verbal communication.

Kathy was young, physically fit, and highly active. She was always on the go, sure-footedly moving around the unit, inside and out. She could run fast when she wanted to and sometimes tried to leap over things in her way. She rarely made eye contact and had repetitive mouth movements that gave her an unusual appearance. Unable to communicate in a 'normal' way, she would bump up against people in her efforts to achieve human connection. This annoyed other residents. The team would always be on the lookout to prevent Kathy from being slapped for getting in someone else's space. Unfortunately, Kathy was drawn to the more difficult-to-get-along-with co-residents, appearing to bump into them to create a bit of fun, before lithely slipping away.

The team took time to collate Kathy's life story, and displayed it in her room, with pictures from across her life enclosed behind Perspex, as Kathy loved to pull everything off the wall. She had been a beautiful young woman, dressed in style, and a delighted young mother of two smiling children. According to her mother, Kathy was a lightning-fast mathematician with a natural aptitude for the computer. She had gone through a messy divorce before the onset of her illness, when she was far too young, confronting her with sadness and loss that she had struggled to accept. Kathy's mother maintained that there was 'more happening in Kathy's mind than people realise'.

Remarkable moments with Kathy helped us better connect her care with her story. One day, out of the blue, she wrote down her name, correctly using her maiden name. We had not seen her do this before; we'd assumed she had lost this capability. She also wrote her children's names, giving them their correct surname, that of her ex-husband. One day, Kathy wrote down the address of the house where she had lived many years before; so, on a trip on the minibus, the team took her for a drive past her old home. She appeared deeply satisfied to have made the trip.

As Bronnie and Justin explored different ways to engage with Kathy, they discovered that she gravitated toward the portable computer stations on wheels that we used for clinical documentation. Not much bothered by service rules, they set Kathy up with a computer to see what she would do. It was amazing. She could type, and always used the correct spelling – we later discovered that she could correct spelling mistakes team members made on notices around the house.

We also discovered that she loved to use a calculator. Bronnie gave her an Etch A Sketch, and, rather than drawing pictures, she would provide the correct answers to sums written out for her.

When Kathy needed to visit the dentist, she was given a dose of medication to ease the anxiety that would understandably escalate with the trip. The drug had a paradoxical effect – the opposite of what we expected to see. Instead of calming down, she sped up. She went for a run around the garden, and was almost impossible to contain. The dentist trip was cancelled. An hour later, to everyone's amazement, Kathy started talking. She spoke fluently, reflecting on issues of life, conflict and sadness. The context of the conversation was not entirely clear, but the fact she had retained the ability to use language was unmistakable. The effect of the medication eventually wore off, and Kathy returned to her usual presentation. There were several similar episodes, and we went through cautious discussions with Kathy's mother, debating options for other treatment trials to see if we could achieve a more sustained 'awakening' of Kathy's language. Frustratingly, Kathy's 'unlocking' came at the cost of rampant motor activity, which, at its worst, resulted in a nasty fall. Nonetheless, the take-home message was loudly proclaimed: we had to remain curious, seek discoveries, and take none of the people in our care for granted.

It is easy to make assumptions about people living with dementia. I learnt from Kathy that what we see on the surface can conceal extraordinary capabilities waiting to be discovered.

I arrived at Northgate House following three weeks of annual leave. Kathy was taking a quiet moment, sitting in the sun with her Etch A Sketch. To my shame, I didn't speak with her, being distracted by a much noisier person who had demanded my attention. A little while later, I moved on, and Justin came chasing after me, holding Kathy's Etch A Sketch.

'Look!' he said, 'Look what she wrote!'

I looked down at the board and was dumbfounded. Amid some numbers and a few squiggles, there was one word, written neatly and correctly: *Duncan.*

Oh, my goodness,' I gasped, 'Kathy knows me. She knows my name.'

How easily I had assumed that I was of limited importance in Kathy's world just because she could not speak and only communicated by occasionally bumping into me during my regular visits. Each time I arrived after that, I made sure to say hello, irrespective of whether Kathy acknowledged me.

As we grew, learning more about the people we cared for as well as each other, friendships formed. The stories of residents and team members seemed to merge together. After Bronnie received her cancer diagnosis, she was forced to stop working for a time and found herself confronted with existential uncertainty. She desperately missed her engagement with the people she was passionate about, both her colleagues and the people who lived in our care at Northgate House. Just before Christmas, the team wanted to do something special for her. Flowers and a gift just didn't seem right, so they came up with a plan to pay Bronnie a visit at her home, not long before she was due to go into the hospital for surgery. Several team members climbed aboard the Northgate House minibus, taking our resident Kathy with them.

The team arrived at Bronnie's house, and she greeted them at the front gate, pale and unwell but delighted. Within a moment of seeing Bronnie, Kathy was off the bus. Without a word, Kathy wrapped her arms around Bronnie, pushing her face down into her shoulder. It was a rare moment, even more remarkable considering the degree of Kathy's disability. It would have been easy to assume that Kathy would neither have recalled Bronnie nor have been interested in hugging her. And yet there were tears, as sadness, anxiety and joy intermingled in a moment of living. Living with dementia; living with cancer; living with stress and conflict and friendship all at once. Bronnie subsequently said that there had been no more wonderful Christmas moment for her, ever.

❖ ❖ ❖

I could go on and on. There are as many stories to tell as there are people. The lesson here in relation to people living with dementia is significant. But what if we extrapolate this to other services, relationships and contexts? The same principles apply. An appreciation of people's stories can change the way we understand them and how we provide care. The impact of this is bountiful. What we learnt was felt by the people in our care and their families, who joined our community as partners.

And so, our chequered, values-driven team learnt to work together; to be open and flexible; transparent and present; continuously seeking to understand our people more intrinsically; giving things a try – and readjusting and adapting if they didn't work. We reminded ourselves that it was okay to make mistakes, that we just needed to learn from them. Each person's story was the centrepiece in planning their care, which was undertaken with a commitment to see beyond dementia and every other infirmity. And it made all the difference.

19

Burning down and burning out

We all have personal valleys. In late 2019, an unexpected and dark twist in my story occurred, bringing salient lessons in sustainability and living with purpose.

After sneaking up for a while, a profound exhaustion came upon me. After nearly three years of striving in the work of remediation after the Oakden Report, I could not keep it at bay. I had maintained a positive public attitude as I reported our successes and progress on the reform imperatives. I knew we were onto something important, but this created a catch-22 for me. I sincerely believed that the insights offered through the Oakden stories were of profound relevance to all healthcare providers, and to life in general. I knew that we had come a long way, and I stuck to this narrative at every public opportunity. But I also feared that progress might be superficial; that it was fragile and could be undone at the drop of a hat. And if this were to happen, it would undermine the veracity of the insights we had gained. In response to this, I took upon myself an excessive pressure to succeed, in contradiction to the very ideas to which I had committed.

Concurrently, I was concerned that those in the bureaucratic healthcare system around me had not taken what we had learnt to heart. There remained a strong systemic propensity to return to baseline – to cultures characterised by compliance, hierarchical power relationships, anxiety and othering. I was worn out by the strain of swimming upstream in a world where simply fitting into the health service status quo was good enough, provided we were not committing the overt failures of old. My inability to reconcile the various Oakden narratives, my earnest desire to create an oasis of compassionate, counter-cultural caring, and my own vulnerability – all fuelled by fear of failing to fulfil these lofty aspirations – set me up against unrealistic expectations that required unsustainable levels of effort.

In November of 2019 I attended an interstate conference as an invited speaker, to share what we had learnt from Oakden. I presented my session. To my colleagues around me, I appeared fine. But the months of disturbed sleep, continual tension, neglect of physical health and family relationships and, more than anything, the ever-present anxiety that I may not be able to deliver the promised degree of transformation – despite spruiking the story wherever possible – came to a head. I found myself overwhelmed with feelings of panic and hopelessness. I felt like a charlatan. How could I be talking about these ideas and yet be such a mess myself?

The morning after I had spoken at the conference, the physical aches, pains and agitation that had plagued me for months culminated in a wry neck such as I had never experienced before. My eyes watered, and I couldn't concentrate. I made it home from the conference, concealing my tribulations and maintaining a pretence of control. A few days later, via a further turn of events, I had a bladder tumour resected and endured an anxious wait for the biopsy results.

It was a great relief when the results indicated a lesion of low malignant potential. The excruciating neck pain gradually resolved. But I was unable to continue pretending. I had emotionally and physically hit a wall. It was time to take stock.

I was in burnout.

No amount of noble intention could compensate for or deny it. For a long time, I had told myself that I would be fine to keep going, to press onward, and had convinced myself that I was somehow deficient if I could not. Wholeheartedness and hubris held hands within me, like a contradictory couple.

Burnout is an all-too-common problem. Studies suggest that rates of burnout can run between ten and seventy per cent, depending on the discipline.[1] People in caring and service professions appear to be significantly affected, including nurses, midwives, doctors, social workers and teachers. But it is not just caring professions. People working in other sectors, such as banking and finance, also report high levels of work-related stress and burnout.[2]

The costs for individuals and organisations are high. It has been estimated that burnout costs the United States $125–190 (US) billion in healthcare each year.[3] In Australia, workplace stress costs at least $14 (AUD) billion each year.[4] The implications for people's health are substantial, with evidence suggesting an increased hospitalisation risk for mental health and cardiovascular events in the decade following an episode of burnout.[5] One study found that ninety per cent of people with severe burnout symptoms also had other physical and mental health problems, including pain and depression.[6]

Despite this body of evidence, and the experience of many people, there remains confusion, even scepticism, regarding burnout. It becomes too easy to invalidate the experience and make it the sufferer's problem. There is no denying that personal factors contribute to vulnerability to burnout – a tendency to perfectionism, for instance, has been proffered as a predisposing factor. But this is only part of the story. Burnout has implications for workplaces themselves. The research shows that burnout can function as a 'contagious' phenomenon.[7, 8] It tends to spread. This underlines the fact that we cannot separate a conversation about burnout from one about workplace culture and community.

Many workplace cultures subtly encourage staff to manage their working lives in ways that are not healthy or balanced. Have you encountered the phenomenon of the 'busy-off'? Picture yourself stepping into a lift with a colleague you haven't seen for a while. After initial greetings, you end up swapping commentary on how busy you are, how it's impossible to keep up, and how the constant avalanche of demands is relentless. The two of you end up in a not-so-subtle contest over who is carrying the weightier load and having the toughest time of it. Busier is synonymous with better.

Swiping through LinkedIn recently, I came across a colleague bemoaning that too many people in their workplace were 'wearing their burnout like a badge of honour'. In desperation, this colleague declared in a social-media vow of resolution that they would break free of this in the coming year.

When I was working ridiculous hours and wrestling with implacable angst at the height of the Oakden scandal, CEO Jackie Hanson asked me how I was and if I needed anything. It was good that she asked me, and I have no doubt that she was sincerely concerned; she was also experiencing the undue stress of the season, and we shared a strong sense of identification as a result. The problem was that something about the situation made me feel the only right answers were: 'Thank you, I'm fine,' and: 'No, I have everything I need.'

At the time, I struggled to identify exactly what *would* help me, although, in retrospect, I was clearly on a pathway to being *not* fine. Hindsight is a great teacher, and I hope I would respond differently today. How much of this was my perfectionist desire to be okay, to not need help? How much was a subtle cultural pressure; that to ask for an extra resource or admit to not coping was to concede incapacity? Was I storing up points for my next busy-off?

As I look back at my burnout experience, it's obvious that there was a lack of balance in my workload. Some of this was circumstantial and reflected the organisational landscape – everyone was working extended hours and the 'busy-off' was a common phenomenon. And some of it was my own decision-making, driven by a range of motivations. At first, I maintained the energy to keep going, but only for a time. As I became more exhausted, my ability to see things clearly deteriorated.

Also contributing to my burnout were issues around control, reward and values. During the early period after Oakden, I had felt a powerful sense of agency and control. Despite the whirlwind, intense pressure and steep learning curve, it was an agile time. Those of us working together at the centre of the action were able to get things done quickly; for a short while, the normal processes for making decisions, accessing funding, and cutting red tape faded. We had direct access to executive approvals. This changed as life shifted back toward 'business as usual'. The rate of progress slowed. But, to me, the priorities seemed no less obvious, and I became increasingly frustrated by how difficult it was to translate vision into change that would stand the test of time. I felt out of control – but still carried high expectations of success.

A disconnection emerged between my values and aspirations and the landscape around me. It seemed to me that people wanted to forget what had happened at Oakden. They started saying things like, 'Let's not mention the O word again; we need to move on.' We might as well have called the whole thing 'Voldemort'. And then, after my exposure to the machinations of politics and the media, I felt disappointed. I also started to feel angry, bothered by the loss of integrity and nuance in the public narrative and sceptical of departmental rhetoric.

To top things off, around this time, I became embroiled with a particularly difficult-to-work-with family of a person admitted to one of our services. The family could not agree among themselves or with our care team. No matter what the team or I offered, we found ourselves up against complaints and threats of litigation. We were committed to providing compassionate relationship-centred care, informed by an understanding of the person; it was bizarre to be in a situation where the approach that worked with everyone else kept going wrong. I had not encountered such hostility before, and I lost patience. In the soil of exhaustion, the seeds germinating beneath the surface erupted in cynicism and despair. The research suggests that the experience of cynicism is the domain of burnout most likely to influence staff turnover.[9] I felt like a failure and, for the first time since becoming a psychiatrist, I wanted to quit. My mind was overrun with the darkest of thoughts, and for a time, I could not see a chance of improvement.

With things crashing down, I needed to take action. I saw my GP and was honest about what I was feeling. I took some time away from work – not long but just enough to take a breath and re-evaluate. The exhaustion and inability to keep going worked in my favour, compelling me to start changing my expectations. I found that some things were not that difficult to change and, remarkably, changing them did not damage my work outcomes. Simple things helped, like putting in an apology for some work meetings, and no longer obsessively checking my emails at night or on the weekend. These changes created distance from the all-consuming intensity of what was happening at work. This made a difference to my ruminating mind – with improvement in my sleep and mood – and to life at home.

I utilised the Employee Assistance Program, which provided me with access to a psychologist, Clark. We connected well. Over several months, we engaged in a healing conversation. Despite being a psychiatrist, it took the perspective of an objective other to help me make sense of things that I was too close to. Clark helped me see how the hamster wheel I'd been on had allowed burnout to creep up over time. I came to understand how exhaustion, cynicism and inefficacy had infiltrated my thoughts and feelings.[10]

Aspects of my own story emerged spontaneously within our conversations. I recognised and acknowledged interconnections between my unresolved anxiety over my mother's illness and my constant striving within work choices. In one of these conversations, I had a tearful moment of realisation regarding some of my escape fantasies; fuelled by my own fear of the future; struggling with my own mortality.

'Even if I could get away from my work,' I confessed, 'I can't get away from my life.'

Being able to speak into a safe space about how I was feeling, and to have that heard respectfully, enabled me to transition from brittle, raw emotions to a place of greater acceptance. I gradually moved from burned-out depression toward recovery.

Parallel with these conversations, I engaged in my own reflection, reading and contemplation on life, faith and vocation. I found myself asking: how did I get to this place I now find myself in? Where do I go from here? Writing became an important, albeit sometimes torturous, task that helped me process these questions and was part of my recovery.

Clark prompted me to take practical steps. I responded readily. Before climbing aboard the Oakden hamster wheel, I had been committed to the positive management of my diet and exercise. I'd subsequently lost track of this. With a gentle nudge and a renewed commitment to accountability, I started to care for myself again. Lois and I also quarantined time to talk, something else we had lost sight of.

In a spirit of curiosity, I explored other ways to wellness. At the recommendation of a friend who had reported remarkable benefits, I visited a traditional Chinese medicine practitioner. He examined my tongue and immediately shook his head, bemoaning an apparent extreme depletion in my *chi*. I pretended to understand. He prescribed herbal medication – on which I did my homework, recognising the limited science available. My family's verdict was that it did seem to help my recovery.

As a psychiatrist, I was familiar with the literature and evidence supporting the benefits of mindfulness practice. I was also aware of the proliferation of mindfulness-lite apps, downloadable to people's phones and iPads. I had some caution regarding the value of approaches that were not adequately rigorous. Yet my knowledge of mindfulness was purely academic. To address this, I enrolled in a training course for mental health practitioners, which led me through a program of mindfulness-integrated cognitive behavioural therapy with one of Australia's leading mindfulness practitioners. My concerns over rigour were quickly put aside. It was hard work; one of the potential limitations to highly efficacious mindfulness practice is that it is a *discipline* – analogous to committing to regular exercise and a healthy diet. But I found mindfulness practice transformative. One of its primary objectives is to move toward equanimity – a mental state in which we are not buffeted around by reactive emotions, regardless of the challenges we encounter. Mindfulness practice helped me to be more emotionally balanced, despite being challenging to embed in daily routines.

❖❖❖

My personal account of burnout may well seem inconsistent with the compassionate, collaborative, humanised teams and the honouring of people's stories that have been described in this book. Doesn't the fact that I went through burnout while aspiring to the way of working described here suggest that what we were doing – and what I'm advocating for – doesn't work? But my experience of burnout has reinforced for me how important it is to overcome barriers to system and culture change and to translate aspiration into action.

In addition to strategies focused on individual recovery and resilience, burnout requires organisational support. Consideration of shared values, building with integrity, nurturing collaborative communities, and attending to psychological safety in the workplace are protective against burnout. They also support healing when burnout occurs.[11]

I needed to change the intensity of my work for a time, but part of my recovery was also found through relationship with like-valued co-travellers, working with them to achieve better, kinder, more compassionate workplace communities. As I resurfaced from feeling submerged, other people – both colleagues and the people and families we served – restored hope in me that the work was worth it, despite the demands and conflicts that we continued to encounter in the wider organisational landscape.

❖❖❖

There is a call to search deeply into the place from which we work and question our motivations. I first read the work of Parker J. Palmer while in the depth of my depression and burnout and was confronted with an alarming challenge. Palmer boldly declared burnout to be the result of 'violating [one's] own nature in the name of nobility'. Harsh words. He wrote:

Usually regarded as the result of trying to give too much, burnout in my experience results from trying to give what I do not possess – the ultimate in giving too little! Burnout is a state of emptiness, to be sure, but it does not result from giving all I have: it merely reveals the nothingness from which I was trying to give in the first place.[12]

When reading this, I felt the call to self-reflection. Yet, when tempered with self-compassion and grace, the potential to come to a quiet sense of self-awareness, such that we contribute our labour from who we are and what we have, rather than something we pretend to be, offers liberation. Palmer's words helped me understand that moving beyond burnout involves being held in the protective, healing support of community. When we have exhausted our own resources and capacity to give, being in community means that we can trust that 'someone else will be available to the person in need'.[13] No one can achieve the type of change described in this book singlehandedly. We need each other. We need a shared sense of purpose, mutual respect, and an ability to pull together when things are difficult.

I am grateful for my experience of burnout. It offered me the gift of brokenness and an opportunity for learning, growth and change: the benefits of failing. It informed a greater sense of realism, tempered my hubris and compelled humility. Rather than strength and success, the rediscovery of hope and learning to give from what I have, rather than striving from what I have not, have been crucial to my continuing recovery. The disciplines of balance and self-care have been necessary and have included redefining priorities and learning to let go. But being part of a team – a community of people each living with brokenness, but living nonetheless, and giving organically from the life and nature within them – has been most important of all. It is in a story-rich community such as this that hope and meaning are retained.

20

On being story-informed

So, how do we bring all this learning and growing together? What are we left with that makes sense and will remain after the scandal has settled and the public and political impetus for reform has waned?

The co-designed reinventions of culture and care that emerged after the Oakden Report had immediate and local significance. Yet I understand that things don't stay the same. Systems and services evolve and change. Governments come and go. Policies and priorities shift. Leadership changes, and people move on.

There must be something more enduring to learn from this story.

I hope that the lessons arising here, which extend beyond the events surrounding Oakden, make a broader, lasting contribution to delivering better care to older people, and people who experience vulnerability, whatever the cause. These lessons may help other communities solve challenging problems. There is insight in this story regarding the need for well-resourced systems of care for older people and those with complex needs. We should be aware of our shared interest in such investment as inevitable future users of these systems.

There are lessons of relevance for governments, politicians, and executives – people of influence and power within our systems. Change is most effective when approached from the ground up. The best leadership will make the effort to search out, understand and connect with the stories and experiences of people who are the human recipients of high-level systems decisions. To politicians and executives: don't forget to listen and engage. We're really all the same, and rank shouldn't have its usual privileges.[1]

There are also lessons that speak to organisations – particularly those that provide health and social care. At all levels, right through to frontline teams, there is no substitute for working on culture – the living expression of values in action – thinking about *how* we work together, not just *what* we do.

And then, there are lessons we might take to heart on a personal level. If we were all to grapple with these opportunities to learn, the challenges at organisational and systems levels might not be so great. And so, we might ask: What am *I* to do with what I have learnt? What can I hold onto and take with me through life?

❖ ❖ ❖

It is a discomforting privilege to work with older people and people with dementia. A privilege for so many reasons; discomforting because there can be no pretending. There are unavoidable, daily reality checks about the nature of things.

There is a fragile space between the all-too-fleeting vigour of youth and the human frailty we encounter at the end of life. It's fragile because, while we blithely tell ourselves things will stay the same and keep on going, the only guarantee is that they won't. We can optimise our health and wellbeing and that of other people – and this is a noble pursuit – but we can neither stave off the passage of time nor unexpected bends in the road.

For the first two tumultuous years after the release of the Oakden Report, I shared an office and worked in partnership with Jacky, our Nursing Director. The unrelenting system reactivity made those years a painfully stressful experience. But we got things done. We had a chance to make a difference in something important, working on it together. We cried. We were outraged. We argued. Most memorably, we laughed. We laughed and laughed, finding strength in humour. When Jacky moved on to new opportunities in 2019, we remained firm friends.

On being story-informed

Then, in November 2020, out of the blue, Jacky received a diagnosis of non-small-cell lung cancer. Over four months, she rapidly and privately traversed that fragile space between vigour and frailty. She died, leaving her family and hundreds of friends shocked and bereaved. I still miss her and find myself conjuring up the image of her bouncing jauntily through the door of our shared office.

Yet we should not live disabled by fear of the future, and so, in the face of life and loss, we need hope that is more robust than the pretence of bodily permanence. We need to make meaning of our lives.

And this brings me back, again, to the importance of stories: to where we started this book. Stories express meaning. They are humanising. Stories are an antidote to seeing people as 'other' than ourselves. In drawing this book to a close, I want to bring attention back to the power of storytelling and story-listening to connect us with each other. If you take something away from reading this book that changes how you think, live, work and serve, let it be this.

In his book *Being Mortal*, surgeon, thinker and writer Atul Gawande powerfully captured the importance of stories in meaning-making:

In the end, people don't view their life as merely the average of all its moments – which, after all, is mostly nothing much plus some sleep. For human beings, life is meaningful because it is a story. A story has a sense of a whole, and its arc is determined by the significant moments, the ones where something happens.

As we come alongside and are *with* people, our task is to listen, observe and connect with those significant moments that shape the arc of their stories. The 'peaks of joy and valleys of misery', as Gawande put them. Like us, people seek to recognise how their story 'works out as a whole'.[2]

Bringing this together, I think about the idea of '*being story-informed*', built around the central importance of listening to and honouring a person's story. I'm conscious that we don't need another model for providing care, as such. We already have the insights and wisdom of person-centred, relationship-centred, and trauma-informed care.

Alongside these, 'narrative medicine', pioneered by Dr Rita Charon from the University of Columbia, has called for doctors, and other health professionals, to develop 'narrative skills', which involve 'absorbing, interpreting and being moved by the stories of illness'. Charon proposed narrative medicine as a corrective for the dominance of medicine's technical aspects over the human and experiential.

Narrative medicine draws connections between patients' stories and doctors' own evolving life narratives. It also draws on rich learning yielded by a reflective reading of the arts and literature – whether fiction, non-fiction or poetry. Charon pointed out that, by developing 'narrative competence', doctors are better able to 'bear witness' to their patients' stories of suffering, loss and tragedy with courage and generosity, and to tolerate their own inability to answer all the questions and solve the problems.[3]

One of the potential issues with narrative medicine, relevant to our discussion here, is its medical orientation. Dr Josephine Ensign, herself a practitioner of narrative medicine, pointed out that this approach relies on 'an ideal encounter between an empathic physician and a cognitively intact, compliant adult patient'.[4] What does this mean for people who might not fit these parameters; or who are excluded from healthcare because of disadvantage; or who cannot speak for themselves, whatever the reason?

And so, as I have reflected on the stories and experiences you have read about across the pages of this book, I have found this idea of 'being story-informed', helpful in making sense of what I have learnt. It brings together important elements from these other approaches while not being limited to a clinical context. It has relevance for everyone as we make our way in the world.

So how can we frame this in such a way that it helps us translate ideas into active living?

❖❖❖

I think of being story-informed as an **approach** built on the cornerstones of *empathy, compassion* and *equality*. It promotes supportive **attitudes** of *curiosity, humility* and *non-judgement*, which guide the **actions** of *listening, imagining* and *learning*. It's worth exploring these further.

As an **approach**, being story-informed builds on empathy, compassion and equality.

The terms 'sympathy' and 'empathy' are often confused. Helen Riess – a psychiatrist, neuroscientist and leading researcher on empathy – captured the two definitions in her highly recommended book, *The Empathy Effect*:

> *Sympathy can be described as the feeling you have when you look out your window and see someone shivering in the cold rain. You feel bad for this person. Empathy is as if you're going out in the rain and standing next to this person, through your imagination, and experiencing his discomfort and distress as if it were your own.*[5]

In attending to and being informed by another's story we can consider what it might be like to walk in their shoes. In this way, empathy provides the motivational power behind compassion – the impetus to see, feel and *do something* about another human's suffering.

Empathy goes hand-in-hand with a commitment to equality. In simple terms, equality means 'the state of being equal';[6] yet, across our world, there are vast differences in experience, wealth, ability and so on. Clearly, everyone is not equal against these measures. And yet, everyone *is* equal in value and should have equal opportunity to 'make the most of their lives and talents', as the UK Equality and Human Rights Commission states. Further, 'no one should have poorer life chances because of the way they were born, where they come from, what they believe or whether they have a disability'.[7] Commitment to equality can help us celebrate diversity, call out othering, and consider how we reduce differences in power between people.

Empathy, compassion and equality tend to be contagious. By stepping into another's shoes and feeling their pain, we are motivated to demonstrate compassion. This brings a positive experience to others who receive our help or who witness it, who are, in turn, more likely to reciprocate empathy, compassion and kindness – responding to others with the embodiment of equality.

The **attitudes** of being story-informed are curiosity, humility and non-judgement.

Curiosity reflects a desire to learn more about something or someone. It's crucial in overcoming our unconscious biases about people who aren't like us. Rather than jumping to conclusions and writing people off, curiosity prompts us to ask questions and seek to understand, without needing to agree. It encourages us to probe deeper. Diana Renner, of the Uncharted Leadership Institute, wrote that curiosity 'opens us to the world around us. It helps us see again with "fresh eyes" and allows us to make new connections'.[8]

Humility reflects our commitment to equality and serving others. A couple of lines from the Bible encapsulate this for me, from Paul's letters to the churches in Rome and Philippi. To the Romans, he said, 'Don't think you are better than you really are. Be honest in your evaluation of yourselves.'[9]

To the Philippians, he said, 'Don't be selfish; don't try to impress others. Be humble, thinking of others as better than yourselves. Don't look out only for your own interests, but take an interest in others, too.'[10]

It's hard to deny that this is good advice.

Most of us don't even realise we're passing judgement on other people. That colleague who came back too late from lunch – typical! The behaviour of those protesting hooligans from the other end of politics – disgraceful. Cast your mind back to the concept of the fundamental attribution error described in the first pages of this book. Here it is again, driving our tendency to pass judgment and leading us to othering, defining boundaries between others and us with sharp distinction. Yet, if we approach interactions with intentional curiosity and humility, we must also withhold judgement as we seek to appreciate perspectives.

In a podcast, hosted by Nathan Foster, Director of Community Life at the Renovaré Institute in the United States, author Lacy Borgo made a powerful statement: 'It's much easier to judge someone from a distance, [but] it's very difficult to judge up close.'[11]

Coming up close to people through listening to their stories helps us balance differences through finding non-judgemental appreciation of our commonality.

Being story-informed requires **action**. It prompts honing our skills in listening, imagining and learning.

We had a season in the Culture Club at Northgate House where we talked a lot about listening. The team was captivated by the idea that we tend to listen in one of three ways: listening to be right, listening to reply, or listening to learn. More often than not, curious, humble, non-judgemental listening requires engaged conversations where we do very little talking and just tune in to what someone else is telling us about their life – being quiet rather than planning what we will say next.

But what if the person *can't* tell us their story – for instance, if they live with a type of dementia that has caused profound speech impairment? Listening can occur in different ways.[12] At Northgate House, we relied heavily on stories provided by families. We were also able to add rich colour to people's stories via pictures, objects and music. Listening with genuine curiosity in these contexts has been just as important as sitting with another person as they recount their experiences in words.

Dennis McDermott was an acclaimed Australian poet and professor. He contributed profound insight on listening, drawing on his perspective as a Koori man, from Gomeroi Country in New South Wales. He referred to Aboriginal traditions of silence, non-verbal communication and reflection. McDermott proposed that these traditions of 'deep listening' offered ways of 'de-othering' the approach of non-Aboriginal health practitioners working with Aboriginal people. Important in this approach of 'deep listening' was the ability to hold all aspects of the person's story, without pulling away:

> If we're deep listening to someone … we are showing that we are not thrown by their fear, their shame, their guilt, their broken story – we can hear the whole thing.[13]

This is relevant for everyone.

Imagining is not merely an idle state of mind or some sort of daydreaming. It is an active process that is an essential component of empathically hearing a person's story. It is the 'as if' component of empathy that requires deliberation – placing ourselves, through imagination, in someone else's experience as we listen to their story. It enables us to identify with and understand others, even when they are very different to us.

Further, imagining is a critical component of finding a way forward and solving problems. It's part of innovating, creating and envisioning future possibilities. Imagination is vital to inspiring hope.

When working with a person who is in dire circumstances – someone in distress, a person with dementia, or disablement, or someone who is dying – we are not merely looking back on their narrative. Their story is still being written, even at the ending of life. By imagining what might be, what might shift in them or their circumstances to ensure the retention of dignity and meaning, we can help infuse hope into a person's situation.

Gawande understands this well. He has pointed out that the 'most cruel failure' in the treatment of older people, and those who are ill, is in failing to recognise a person's continuing drive for existential significance over blindly prioritising issues of safety and survival. 'The chance to shape one's story,' he states, 'is essential to sustaining meaning in life.'[14]

Imagination is vital in inspiring hope that supports people to have agency over their lives.

Finally, learning is an indispensable, active part of living and working in a story-informed way. It is the product of listening and imagining, of approaching engagement with curiosity and without judgement. It is an active process that requires commitment, fortitude and persistence. It requires courageous self-reflection, being prepared to use insight to address our own deficits – which results in us being more able to meet the needs of others. As people share their stories with us, they gift us the opportunity to learn.

❖❖❖

On being story-informed

In becoming story-informed, most of us need a paradigm shift – like the one Stephen Covey experienced when sitting next to the bereaved young father on the train, as we learnt in the first pages of this book.[15] Robert Coles is a psychiatrist, now in his nineties. In his book, *The Call of Stories*, he described his paradigm shift during the first year of his psychiatric residency, while being mentored by two different senior psychiatrists – Doctors Binger and Ludwig.

Dr Binger was academic and diagnostically focused. The hierarchical nature of the supervision process was quickly established. It was constrained and predictable, but therefore comfortably familiar to Coles, following his experience as a medical student and junior resident. In contrast, Dr Ludwig was hard of hearing, affable and eccentric. Supervision was fluid and unpredictable and far more disconcerting for the young Dr Coles.

Coles recounted an experience where he turned up to supervision feeling uncertain and struggling to make sense of his 'cases'. He felt like he was a patient turning up for therapy. Dr Ludwig sensed this disruption of Coles' readiness to learn and instead of their normal process, took the opportunity to tell Dr Coles a 'story'.

Dr Ludwig recounted the narrative of a woman – his patient – who was paralysed by anxiety. He described all sorts of captivating details about her life and what was important to her. Then, suddenly, her life was interrupted by a terrible car accident. Dr Coles was horrified, taken aback. He was completely caught up in the story of a person who was real, with a name, a life. He had completely forgotten that this was a clinical history he was hearing.

Cole's words capture the next moments the best:

'I have told you a story,' the doctor said. Nothing more. I waited for an amplification in vain. It was my turn. I responded to the storyteller, not the doctor, the psychiatrist, the supervisor: 'What happened?' I was a little embarrassed at the sound in my own ears of those two words, for I felt I ought to have asked a shrewd psychological question. But Dr Ludwig said he was glad I'd asked the question I did. Then he told me 'what happened'.

Afterward, there was a different kind of silence in the room, for I was thinking about what I'd heard, and he was remembering what he had experienced. Finally, he gave me a brief lecture that I would hear in my head many times over the next three decades:

'The people who come to see us bring us their stories. They hope they tell them well enough so that we understand the truth of their lives. They hope we know how to interpret their stories correctly. We have to remember that what we hear is their story.'

He stopped there, waited for me to speak. But I had nothing to say.[16]

After this, rather than approaching his patients with the psychiatrist's hovering intent to clarify a diagnosis, propose a formulation and determine a therapeutic agenda, Coles began, first and foremost, to listen and connect. This is the heart of being story-informed.

❖ ❖ ❖

I'm aware this all sounds idealistic. It might seem saccharine – a bonkers utopia for Pollyannas and ponies. It'd be difficult *not* to have some scepticism. We are exploring a more ideal way of living and working here – one that addresses some of the core cultural problems in healthcare and in many other settings. There are many challenges. There must be space to make mistakes, to fall short of expectations, to pick ourselves up and try again. It's worth embracing the aspiration with a healthy dose of humour and kind-hearted self-deprecation. This can bring realism and balance to a potentially zealous intensity that might be off-putting.

Should you find yourself in the mood for a distracting dive down a YouTube rabbit hole, allow me to recommend a classic sketch from the comedy team at *Saturday Night Live*. It features the remarkably talented Kristen Wiig as the NBC's *Today* show host Kathie Lee Gifford. Wiig's portrayal of Gifford is merciless. After a crass interaction with her co-anchor, Hoda Kotb, whom she continuously mocks and ridicules, Gifford (Wigg) launches into a song she has written: 'Everyone has a Story'.

It's the most ridiculous, clichéd tripe. In the middle of the song, she fires a shot at her co-anchor, singing, 'Hoda has a story. And Hoda's story is boring!'

Shortly after this, the special guests on the show, the legendary pop group The Black Eyed Peas, have had enough; they race onto the set to throw themselves at Gifford, wrestling her to the ground. The sketch ends with Gifford clambering to her feet to finish her song, hair bedraggled and a bottle of Chardonnay in hand.[17]

As I laugh hysterically at this sketch, I am conscious of the irony.

Off I go to work the next day, reminding myself and others that everyone has a story, and that our task is to listen, connect, learn and offer help. There is a risk that the sentiments here could be seen as feel-good platitudes that are unlikely to be applied in the real world. But I don't see it this way. Being aspirational does not negate the integrity of intention. Nor does striving to find a language of hope trivialise the real pain people experience in their lives. Being story-informed doesn't require us to get everything right. It asks us to be more reflective and shift our perspective.

❖❖❖

On the bad days, working in public mental health services can feel like doing business in the domain of human misery. It can be hard.

Not long ago I covered a shift in a local emergency department, the realm of rapid-fire assessments and determinations for complex problems. Nearing the end of a busy day, a young man was brought in from a local prison for mental health assessment. I received a brief handover before I went to see him.

He had been born with a mild intellectual disability into a home where he was subjected to physical, emotional and sexual abuse. His brushes with the law commenced when he was still a child and escalated through his young adult years, including spells in prison with convictions for assault, robbery and drug offences. He had spent so much time incarcerated that he struggled to sustain a life in the community.

I could hear his distress, anger and defensiveness from down the corridor before I arrived at his room. I bumped into the preceding doctor; he was bidding a hasty retreat, with verbal insults being hurled after him through the door.

'He's okay physically,' the doctor said as he passed me in the corridor.

As I entered the room, I noticed the contusion on his forehead where he had been banging his head against a Perspex screen in his cell. His bare feet were dry, cracked and embedded with dirt. He wore nothing but shorts, and a hospital gown draped around his upper body, which was slender but tensely muscular.

Before I had a chance to say anything, he yelled at me, hurling the most nefarious insults, to ensure I knew where I stood with him. Suddenly, he attempted to launch himself toward me from the barouche. He was handcuffed and chained in place, but such was his aggressive determination that the whole contraption lifted from the floor and threatened to tip over. My heart skipped several beats. I contemplated what might have happened had he not been restrained – as is the plight of a prisoner in hospital.

I quietly let him know that I'd be back in ten minutes to try again.

On my second attempt, we progressed with a conversation. He talked about his personal needs, and his perceptions of several female prison officers. He used such vulgar, dehumanising words to describe the officers. It was confronting. He appeared to have no sense of what it might be to speak respectfully about another human being. I was able to make enough of an assessment to be confident that, while his difficulties were manifold and complex, there was no hospital treatment, mental health or otherwise, that would help him that day. My hands felt empty, and my heart heavy with the conundrum in front of me.

I found myself engaged in an internal dialectic. He was not a likeable young man. He was surly, angry, hostile and aggressive. There was an element of genuine danger and, such was his difficulty managing his emotions and behaviour, in different circumstances I would not have been safe. He appeared unable to shift beyond a primitive conceptualisation of other people existing only relative to his needs and efforts to ensure survival.

Yet, at the same time, I had a repeated thought: This young man has his own story.

I knew enough to understand that he had been afforded no advantages and few opportunities. His early attachments to family and care providers had been utterly disrupted. He had started life with developmental disadvantage compounded by poverty and social chaos. His presentation in the emergency department that afternoon had been a long time coming.

Having no service to offer him, I returned him to the custody of the two prison officers who had accompanied him to the hospital. I struggled to reconcile my contradictory responses to him. Alarmed, frightened, confronted – yet deeply sad. I cautiously acknowledged his present situation as the consequence of behaviours, while also recognising a mosaic, circumstantial, lifelong narrative that accounted for why he had come to be there that day. Standing in that awkward, conflicted place, I was leaning into what it means to be story-informed on a tough day.

Talking to this young man, I had made a particular effort to call him by his name. To speak with kindness and respect. I chose to imagine that, somehow, he might get support that would turn his life around – he had referred positively to his interaction with one of the correctional services psychologists.

Just maybe …, I thought to myself.

I chose to maintain hope on his behalf.

❖ ❖ ❖

I recently heard the story of a couple in their nineties, Stefan and Mara. Their situation was heartbreaking. They had been together for over seventy years, having been sweethearts from childhood. Their families had been neighbours in Romania in the 1930s. They had endured hardship and trauma. Marrying in their late teens, they had escaped war-torn Europe for a new life in Australia, like so many others. They had worked hard, building a wholesome life together. They had a daughter, Sofia. She had grown up, a first-generation Aussie, with new opportunities and expectations. She'd married, and Stefan and Mara had delighted in their grandchildren.

As the years passed, Stefan and Mara had both taken steps toward the frailty that comes to everyone in the end. Mara was diagnosed with dementia. She progressively forgot more and moved less. Circumstances conspired and they could no longer live in their small home. Both were placed in a residential aged care facility. After seventy years in constant companionship, their concessional status meant that they did not have the resources to access a couple's room. They were accommodated on different floors. Mara was lost and alone, unable to make sense of where Stefan had gone. Stefan was devastated.

It is a remarkable thing that experiences considered traumatic at earlier stages of the lifespan – such as forced relocation, separation from loved ones and the acquiring of a disability – are frequently dismissed as 'normal' and 'expected' for older people. They are every bit as traumatic.[18] This was the experience of Stefan and Mara.

Sofia began to advocate, seeking to ease her parents' distress. She appealed to the facility.

'Our couples' rooms are all filled,' she was told, 'there's nothing we can do.'

Her advocacy turned to agitation. She argued desperately for their mental health.

'In seventy years, they've never been apart,' she pleaded. 'They're becoming depressed – you can't let this happen to them!'

Sofia wrote a letter to her local member of parliament. The local member wrote a letter to the Federal minister. The minister wrote back, expressing sympathy but explaining that he could do nothing to help – it was up to the aged care provider. The sympathy seemed hollow. The local member forwarded the letter to Sofia. Coming from the other side of politics, he was quick to point out that this was both disappointing and typical of such a government. He then closed the case with a similarly hollow thud.

On being story-informed

When Stefan and Mara's story crossed my path, I was outraged and saddened. My first thought was that we could surely do better at finding a solution to what seemed a relatively simple problem. It is the business of an aged care provider to hold people's stories with dignity and honour. How could they not see that it was not okay to tell a couple in the last days of their lives, after seventy years of togetherness, that they must suddenly adapt to a life of separation? There was a disturbing absence of story-informed kindness and care.

Sofia contacted the local Aged Rights Advocacy Service, persisting with her very reasonable request that her parents be brought together. She knew that in the deep hours of the night, the only soothing balm for their shared distress was each other's presence.

But the weight of grief, shrouded in a shadowy veil of confusion and unfamiliar surroundings took its toll on Mara. She lost interest in being out of bed, then stopped eating. A short while later, with the matter still unresolved, she died. Stefan remained broken-hearted.

And then, a week later, a picture of another couple, Margaret and Derek, appeared on my social media newsfeed – both ninety-one, married for seventy years, sweethearts since the age of fourteen. It was like a parallel universe.

Margaret and Derek had been admitted to separate NHS hospitals in the UK with their own complications of frailty. In hospital, Margaret contracted COVID. The doctors and nurses quickly recognised the limitations confronting them. In the face of the intensity and widespread trauma carried by NHS staff, compassion prevailed. Derek was moved from one hospital to another so that he could be with his wife. Derek subsequently caught COVID too.

'To be honest,' his daughter reported, 'he probably wouldn't have had it any other way. There was no way he wasn't going to go and see her.'[19]

After ninety-one years of living, seventy years of love and companionship, five children, eleven grandchildren and four great-grandchildren, Derek and Margaret slipped beyond life within three days of each other. Their last photograph, taken in hospital by their daughter, is poignant, beautiful and heart wrenching. With hospital beds jammed up against each other, Derek and Margaret can be seen reaching out to one another, their four hands intertwined. It is clear that Margaret, weakened and frail with exhaustion, drew comfort from Derek's touch. Derek's face, overwhelmed by emotion, welled up with love and tears, is the focus of the image. In the wake of the pandemic that battered the NHS, the story of these two people was honoured. The foundations of empathy and compassion remained intact.

By being story-informed in work, relationships and life, we see beyond the immediate and can consider a whole narrative with its twists and turns, traumas and triumphs. We recognise that, in the end, what everyone craves is human connection. We need each other. We need to know that we are valued and that our lives have meaning. At the centre of everyone's story is a need for compassion, hope and humanity – for love. It's simple but true, and every one of us can bring something of this to our part of the world each day.

Notes

Once upon a time ...

1   Bochner, A. & Ellis, C. (2016). *Evocative autoethnography: Writing lives and telling stories.* Routledge.

2   Burton, R. (2013, April 22). *Where science and story meet: We make sense of the world through stories – A deep need rooted in our brains.* https://nautil.us/issue/0/the-story-of-nautilus/where-science-and-story-meet.

3   Greenfield, S. (Speaker). (2011, December 11). Susan Greenfield on storytelling. [video podcast]. https://vimeo.com/33716283.

4   Koenig, J. (2013) 'Sonder.' *The dictionary of obscure sorrows.* https://www.dictionaryofobscuresorrows.com/post/23536922667/sonder.

5   Francis, R. (2013). *Report of the Mid Staffordshire NHS Foundation Trust public inquiry.* The Stationery Office.

6   *ibid.*

7   Groves, A., Thomson, D., McKellar, D., & Proctor, N. (2017). *The Oakden Report.* South Australian Department of Health.

8   Carnell, K. and Paterson, R. (2017). *Review of national aged care quality regulatory processes.* Australian Government Department of Health. https://www.health.gov.au/health-topics/aged-care/aged-care-reforms-and-reviews/review-of-national-aged-care-quality-regulatory-processes. Accessed 25 September 2021.

9   Lander, B.T. (2018). *Oakden: A shameful chapter in South Australia's history.* Independent Commissioner Against Corruption.

10 Commonwealth of Australia. (2021). *Royal Commission into Aged Care Quality and Safety. Final Report: Care, Dignity and Respect.* https://agedcare.royalcommission.gov.au/sites/default/files/2021-03/final-report-volume-1_0.pdf

11 Royal Commission into violence, abuse, neglect and exploitation of people with disability. https://disability.royalcommission.gov.au. Accessed 25 September 2021.

12 Hello My Name Is. (2021). *A message from Kate about the campaign.* https://www.hellomynameis.org.uk.

13 Feltman, C., Hammond, S.A., Hammond, R., Marshall, A. & Bendis, K. (2009). *The thin book of trust: An essential primer for building trust at work.* Thin book publishing.

14 Dunn, D.S. (2011). 'Situations matter: Teaching the Lewinian link between social psychology and rehabilitation psychology.' *History of Psychology,* 4(4), 405–411.

15 Langdridge, D. & Butt, T. (2004). 'The fundamental attribution error: A phenomenological critique'. *British Journal of Social Psychology,* 43(3), 357–369.

16 Rice, M. (2015). 'Unconscious bias and its effect on healthcare leadership'. The Guardian.com. https://www.theguardian.com/healthcare-network/2015/may/19/healthcare-leadership-best-practice-unconscious-bias.

17   Covey, S.R. (1989). *The seven habits of highly effective people: Restoring the character ethic.* Simon and Schuster.

18   Simpson, M. (2019). 'Who is Julie Bailey? The whistleblowing daughter who exposed Stafford Hospital scandal at centre of tonight's TV drama'. *Stoke on Trent Live.* https://www.stokesentinel.co.uk/news/stoke-on-trent-news/jule-bailey-stafford-cure-nhs-3660502.

19   Bochner, A. & Ellis, C. (2016). *Evocative autoethnography: Writing lives and telling stories.* Routledge.

20   Working Narratives. (2013). *What is public narrative and how can we use it?* https://workingnarratives.org/article/public-narrative/.

1   When I become the other

1   Barter-Godfrey, S. & Taket, A. (2009). 'Othering, marginalisation and pathways to exclusion in health'. In A. Taket, B.R. Crisp, A. Nevill, G. Lamaro, M. Graham & S. Barter-Godfrey (Eds.), *Theorising Social Exclusion.* (1st edn, pp. 166–172). Routledge.

2   De Beauvoir, S. (1972). *The second sex.* (H.M. Parshley, Trans.). Penguin. (1949).

3   Okolie, A.C. (2003) 'Identity: Now you don't see it; Now you do'. *Identity: An International Journal of Theory And Research,* 3(1), 1–7.

4   Orrell, J. & Ash, J. (2019). 'Otherness in practice (in the health professions)'. In J. Higgs, S. Cork & D. Horsfall. (Eds.), *Challenging Future Practice Possibilities* (pp. 219–228). Brill Sense.

5   Bauman, Z. (1991). *Modernity and ambivalence.* Polity.

6   BEL Communications. (2019, October 18). 'Riding the wave of the Silver Tsunami: Understanding the link between families and health in old age.' University of Queensland, Australia, Faculty of Business, Economics & Law. https://bel.uq.edu.au/article/2019/10/riding-wave-silver-tsunami-understanding-link-between-families-and-health-old-age.

7   McKellar, D., Ng, F. & Chur-Hansen, A. (2016). 'Is death our business? Philosophical conflicts over the end-of-life in old age psychiatry'. *Aging & Mental Health,* 20(6), 583–593.

8   Greenberg, T. (2009, August 11). 'The invisible years: Thoughts on why the elderly become invisible.' *Psychology Today.* https://www.psychologytoday.com/us/blog/21st-century-aging/200908/the-invisible-years?amp.

9   Kitwood, T. (1997). *Dementia reconsidered: The person comes first.* Open University Press.

10   Kirsnan, L., Kosiol J., Golenko, X., Radford, K., Fitzgerald, A. & Cartmel, J. (2020). 'Discovering the benefits of intergenerational learning'. *Australian Journal of Dementia Care,* 8(6), 23–26.

11   Boland, M., Powell, T. and Lux, D. (Executive Producers). (2017). *Old people's home for 4 year olds* [Documentary]. CPL Productions.

12   Cuell, D. (Executive Producer). (2019). *Old people's home for 4 year olds* [Documentary]. Endemol Shine Australia.

2   I'll like you for always

1   Kitching, D. (2015). 'Depression in dementia'. *Australian Prescriber,* 38(6), 209–2011.

2   Muliyala, K. & Varghese, M. (2010). 'The complex relationship between depression and dementia'. *Annals of Indian Academy of Neurology,* 13(S), 69–73.

3   Feast, A., Orrell, M., Charlesworth, G., Melunsky, N., Poland, F., & Moniz-Cook, E. (2016). 'Behavioural and psychological symptoms in dementia and the challenges for family carers: Systematic review'. *British Journal of Psychiatry,* 208(5), 429–434.

Notes

4   Macaulay, S. (2018). 'The broken lens of BPSD: Why we need to rethink the way we label the behavior of people who live with Alzheimer Disease'. *Journal of the American Medical Directors Association*, 19(2), 177–180.

5   Martinez-Clavera, C., James, S., Bowditch, E. and Kuruvilla, T. (2017). 'Delayed-onset post-traumatic stress disorder symptoms in dementia'. *Prog. Neurol. Psychiatry*, 21(3), 26–31.

6   Breen, N., Caine, D., & Coltheart, M. (2001). 'Mirrored-self misidentification: Two cases of focal onset dementia'. *Neurocase*, 7(3), 239–254.

7   Commonwealth of Australia. (2021). Royal Commission into Aged Care Quality and Safety. Final Report: Care, Dignity and Respect. https://agedcare.royalcommission.gov.au/sites/default/files/2021-03/final-report-volume-1_0.pdf

8   Gott, M., Ibrahim, A.M., Binstock, R.H. (2011). 'The disadvantaged dying: ageing, ageism and palliative care provision for older people in the UK'. In M. Gott, & C. Ingleton (Eds.), *Living with ageing and dying: international perspectives on end of life care for older people* (pp. 52–62). Oxford University Press.

3   Jeans and genes

1   Dharmadasa, T., Henderson, R.D., Talman, P.S., Macdonell, R.A., Mathers, S., Schultz, D.W., Needham, M., Zoing, M., Vucic, S., & Kiernan, M.C. (2017). 'Motor neurone disease: Progress and challenges'. *Medical Journal of Australia*, 206(8), 357–362.

2   World Health Organisation. (December 9, 2020). *The top 10 causes of death*. https://www.who.int/news-room/fact-sheets/detail/the-top-10-causes-of-death.

3   Australian Institute of Health and Welfare. (2021). *Deaths in Australia*. https://www.aihw.gov.au/reports/life-expectancy-death/deaths-in-australia/contents/leading-causes-of-death. Accessed 25 September 2021.

4   Alzheimer's Society. (2016). *Genetics of dementia. Factsheet 405LP*. https://www.alzheimers.org.uk/sites/default/files/pdf/factsheet_genetics_of_dementia.pdf. Accessed 25 September 2021.

5   Luty, A., Kwok, J., Thompson, E., Blumbergs, P., Brooks, W., Loy, C., Dobson-Stone, C., Panegyres, P., Hecker, J., Nicholson, G., Halliday, G. & Schofield, P. (2008). 'Pedigree with frontotemporal lobar degeneration – motor neuron disease and Tar DNA binding protein-43 positive neuropathology: genetic linkage to chromosome 9'. *BMC Neurology*, 8(32). https://doi.org/10.1186/1471-2377-8-32. Accessed 9 November 2021.

6   Alzheimer's Society UK. (2016) *Genetics of Dementia, Factsheet 405LP*. https://www.alzheimers.org.uk/sites/default/files/pdf/factsheet_genetics_of_dementia.pdf. Accessed 25 September 2021.

7   Frankl, V.E. (1984). *Man's search for meaning: An introduction to logotherapy*. Simon & Schuster.

4   Changing lanes

1   Palmer, P.J. (2000). *Let your life speak: Listening for the voice of vocation*. Jossey-Bass.

2   Sarton, M. (1974). 'Now I become myself', in *Collected Poems, 1930–1973*.

3   Parsons, S. (2014, June 22). *Hubris Syndrome. Surviving Church*. http://survivingchurch.org/2014/06/22/hubris-syndrome/.

4   Carson, B., & Murphey, C.B. (1996). *Think big: Unleashing your potential for excellence*. Zondervan Pub. House.

5   Garber, S. (2014). *Visions of vocation: Common grace for the common good*. InterVarsity Press.

6 On the brink

1 Lander, B.T. (2018). *Oakden: A shameful chapter in South Australia's history.* Independent Commissioner Against Corruption.

2 *ibid.*

7 When the story is told

1 Stafrace, S. & Lilly, A. (2008) *Report on the Review of the Makk and McLeay Nursing Home.* SA Health, Department of Health and Ageing.

2 Bruises on Bob Spriggs' legs (Photo). (2017). ABC News. https://www.abc.net.au/news/2017-04-05/bruises-on-bob-spriggs-legs/8419744?nw=0. Accessed 25 September 2021.

3 Langberg, A. (2018). 'Families of Oakden victims for justice and change but they've paid a high price'. *Advertiser.* https://www.adelaidenow.com.au/news/south-australia/families-of-oakden-victims-fought-for-justice-and-change-but-theyve-paid-a-high-price-for-it/news-story/b2b04179a7464fc45399a737165c352f. Accessed 25 September 2021.

4 El-Khoury, C. (2017). 'Oakden abuse victim's wife tells of heartache, frustration amplified by assault'. *ABC Radio National.* https://www.abc.net.au/news/2017-05-20/oakden-abuse-victims-wife-tells-of-heartache/8536822 Accessed 25 September 2021.

5 Jones, E. (2017). 'Family of Ermanno Serpo tell of mistreatment at Oakden Older Persons' Mental Health Facility'. *Advertiser.* https://www.adelaidenow.com.au/news/south-australia/family-of-ermanno-serpo-tell-of-mistreatment-at-oakden-older-persons-mental-health-facility/news-story/3ee7c69d4b12e09fe0ea0a9eae3c4c03. Accessed 25 September 2021.

8 Stories of place and time

1 Cohen, A., Patel, V. & Minas, H. (2013). 'A brief history of global mental health'. In: M.J. Prince, A. Cohen, H. Minas, & V. Patel (Eds.), *Global mental health: Principles and practice* (pp. 3–26). Oxford University Press.

2 Assal, F. (2019). 'History of Dementia.' *Frontiers of neurology and neuroscience, 44,* 118–126. https://doi.org/10.1159/000494959

3 Payne, C. (2009). *Asylum: Inside the closed world of state mental hospitals.* MIT Press.

4 Goldney, R. (2007). 'Lessons from history: The first 25 years of psychiatric hospitals in South Australia'. *Australasian Psychiatry,* 15(5) pp. 368–371.

5 Bell, M. (2003). 'From the 1870s to the 1970s: The changing face of public psychiatry in South Australia'. *Australasian Psychiatry,* 11(1) pp. 80–86.

6 Buob, D. (2017, July 17) Glenside Hospital – Then and Now. https://www.burnsidehistory.org.au/meeting/glenside-hospital-now/.

9 Culture, contingents and contradictions

1 Manley, K., Sanders, K., Cardiff, S., & Webster, J. (2011). 'Effective workplace culture: the attributes, enabling factors and consequences of a new concept'. *International Practice Development Journal,* 1(2), pp. 1–29.

2 Coyle, D. (2018). *The culture code: The secrets of highly successful groups.* Random House, London.

3 Groves, A., Thomson, D., McKellar, D., & Proctor, N. (2017). *The Oakden Report.* South Australian Department of Health.

4 Bowman, C., Ronch, J., & Madjaroff, G. (2010). *The power of language to create culture.* https://www.edu-catering.com/yahoo_site_admin/assets/docs/Rothschild_funded_The_Power_of_Language_to_Create_Culture.5595952.pdf

Notes

5   Opie, R. (2018). 'Oakden nursing home staff did not feed elderly residents if they were difficult, inquest told.' *ABC News*. https://www.abc.net.au/news/2018-02-27/oakden-residents-underfed-emaciated-inquest-hears/9490432. Accessed 25 September 2021.

6   Opie, R. (2017). 'Oakden nursing home psychologist "traumatised" by staff actions.' *ABC News*. https://www.abc.net.au/news/2017-06-06/oakden-nursing-home-psychologist-traumatised-by-staff-actions/8593886. Accessed 25 September 2021.

7   Lander, B.T. (2018). *Oakden: A shameful chapter in South Australia's history.* Independent Commissioner Against Corruption.

8   Golding, W. (2003). *Lord of the flies: 50th anniversary edition* (50th edn). Penguin Books.

10   A steep and strenuous climb

1   Garber, S. (2014). *Visions of vocation: Common grace for the common good.* Intervarsity Press.

2   Carnell, K. and Paterson, R. (2017). *Review of national aged care quality regulatory processes.* Australian Government Department of Health. https://www.health.gov.au/health-topics/aged-care/aged-care-reforms-and-reviews/review-of-national-aged-care-quality-regulatory-processes. Accessed 25 September 2021.

3   Schein, E.H. (1996). 'Kurt Lewin's change theory in the field and in the classroom: Notes toward a model of managed learning'. *Systems Practice*, 9(1), 27–47.

4   Edmondson, A. (2018). *The fearless organization: Creating psychological safety in the workplace for learning, innovation and growth.* Wiley.

5   Lachance, C.C., Jurkowski, M.P., Dymarz, A.C., Robinovitch, S.N., Feldman, F., Laing, A.C., & Mackey, D.C. (2017). 'Compliant flooring to prevent fall-related injuries in older adults: A scoping review of biomechanical efficacy, clinical effectiveness, cost-effectiveness, and workplace safety'. *PloS one*, 12(2), e0171652. https://doi.org/10.1371/journal.pone.0171652

6   Lane, S. (presenter). (2016). 'Secret camera captures nursing home "suffocation".' *7.30 with Leigh Sales*. https://www.abc.net.au/7.30/secret-camera-captures-nursing-home-suffocation/7659690. Accessed 12 September 2021.

11   Politicians and persuasion

1   Washington, D. (2017). 'Who do you trust: Weatherill or the ICAC?' *InDaily*. https://indaily.com.au/opinion/2017/06/01/trust-weatherill-icac/. Accessed 25 September 2021.

2   9News. (2017). 'SA Parliament rejects public ICAC hearings.' https://amp.9news.com.au/article/dca937b9-2271-4079-86dc-4f41452efe98. Accessed 25 September 2021.

3   Landers, B.T. (2018). *Oakden: A shameful chapter in South Australia's history.* Independent Commissioner Against Corruption.

4   *ibid.*

5   Weatherill, J. (2018). *South Australian government response to the Independent Commissioner Against Corruption's Report Oakden: A shameful chapter in South Australia's history.* Government of South Australia.

6   7News Adelaide [Video] 28 February 2018. 'Oakden scandal: Jay Weatherill responds to ICAC's scathing report.' https://www.facebook.com/7NEWSAdelaide/videos/1870999419597371. Accessed 25 September 2021.

7   Harmsen, N. (2018, February 28). 'SA Premier "deeply sorry" after Oakden ICAC reports five individuals for maladministration.' https://www.abc.net.au/news/2018-02-28/icac-report-on-oakden-aged-care-home-released/9492008. Accessed 25 September 2021.

8   Landers, B.T. (2018). *Oakden: A shameful chapter in South Australia's history.* Independent Commissioner Against Corruption.

9   7News Adelaide [Video] 28 February 2018. 'Oakden scandal: Jay Weatherill responds to ICAC's scathing report.' https://www.facebook.com/7NEWSAdelaide/videos/1870999419597371. Accessed 25 September 2021.

12   Media and messaging

1   Hunt, J. (2016). *From a blame culture to a learning culture.* gov.uk. https://www.gov.uk/government/speeches/from-a-blame-culture-to-a-learning-culture.

2   James, C. (2017). 'Time to come clean on nursing home scandal.' *Advertiser.* https://www.adelaidenow.com.au/news/opinion/colin-james-whos-to-blame-over-oakden-nursing-home-scandal/news-story/93508bb824dd625381b18318cf53f4c8

3   Mediaweek. (2018, June 4). 'SA media awards: ABC's Angelique Donnellan named SA journalist of the year.' mediaweek.com.au. https://www.mediaweek.com.au/2018-sa-media-awards-winners-angelique-donnellan/

4   Dornin, T. (2019, February 12). 'Widow recalls husband's horror death.' *Bulletin.* https://www.themorningbulletin.com.au/news/oakden-whistleblower-fronts-royal-commission-into-/3645296/

5   *Advertiser.* (2018, March 1). https://victoriarollison.files.wordpress.com/2018/03/1-mar.jpg.

6   Coê, C. (2018, September 16). 'One of Australia's greatest disgraces': PM Scott Morrison announces royal commission into aged care sector. *Daily Mail, Australia.* https://www.dailymail.co.uk/news/article-6172345/One-Australias-greatest-disgraces-Scott-Morrison-calls-commission-aged-care-sector.html.

7   Holderhead, S. (2017, April 28). 'Mental Health Minister Leesa Vlahos went on two-week European tour and Tunarama festival before visiting Oakden aged care centre.' *Advertiser.* https://www.adelaidenow.com.au/news/south-australia/mental-health-minister-leesa-vlahos-went-on-twoweek-european-tour-and-tunarama-festival-before-visiting-oakden-aged-care-centre/news-story/2fb6bdbaf654b8faee7906f95bbc3ce2

8   Society of Professional Journalists. (2014). *SPJ Code of Ethics.* https://www.spj.org/ethicscode.asp.

9   Macquarie Dictionary. (2021, February 4). 'The Macquarie Dictionary word of the decade winner is …' *Macquarie Dictionary Blog.* https://www.macquariedictionary.com.au/blog/article/780/

10   McGrath, R. (Speaker). (2018) Television advertisement authorised by Liberal Party Adelaide.

11   https://www.facebook.com/7NEWSAdelaide/videos/2025462884151023

12   Langberg, A. (2018, July 5). 'Three years accreditation for Northgate House that replaced condemned Oakden nursing home'. *Advertiser.* https://www.adelaidenow.com.au/news/south-australia/three-years-accreditation-for-northgate-house-that-replaced-condemned-oakden-nursing-home/news-story/440b03e334037f7bdde73ceb42b3f056

13   What matters most

1   Penney, D. & Stastny, P. (2009). *The lives they left behind: Suitcases from a state hospital attic.* Bellevue Literary Press.

2   *ibid.*

14   Co-design and compassion

1   Charlton, J.I. (1998). *Nothing about us without us: Disability oppression and empowerment.* University of California Press.

2   Blomkamp, E. (2018). 'The promise of co-design for public policy'. *Australian Journal of Public Administration*, 77(4), pp. 729-743. doi:10.1111/1467–850.

3   SA Health. (2018). *The 'Oakden Report' Response. The work of the Oakden Response Plan Oversight Committee.* South Australian Government. https://www.sahealth.sa.gov.au/wps/wcm/connect/dd70238c-ac1d-4b23-85fb-670479278d79/Oakden+Response+Report_FINAL+s.pdf?MOD=AJPERES&CACHEID=ROOTWORKSPACE-dd70238c-ac1d-4b23-85fb-670479278d79-nwLgRKQ. Accessed 25 September 2021.

4   SA Health. (2018). *Response to the final report of the Oakden Report Response Plan Oversight Committee.* South Australian Government. https://www.sahealth.sa.gov.au/wps/wcm/connect/f04c4d6a-c7cc-4ed7-a4da-7cbcae4af049/Oakden+Response+Report_FINAL.pdf?MOD=AJPERES&CACHEID=ROOTWORKSPACE-f04c4d6a-c7cc-4ed7-a4da-7cbcae4af049-nwLHCvJ. Accessed 25 September 2021.

5   McKellar, D. & Hanson, J. (2020). 'Codesigned framework for organisational culture reform in South Australian older mental health services after the Oakden Report.' *Australian Health Review*, 44(6), pp. 862-866. doi: 10.1071/AH18211.

6   Harper, D. (2021). 'Compassion (n).' *Online etymology dictionary.* https://www.etymonline.com/word/compassion.

7   Worline, M.C. & Dutton, J.E. (2017). *Awakening compassion at work: The quiet power that elevates people and organizations.* Berret-Koehler.

8   Kitwood, T.M. (1997). *Dementia reconsidered: The person comes first.* Open University Press.

9   Edinburgh Napier University. (2012). *Leadership in compassionate care programme executive summary.* https://www.napier.ac.uk/~media/worktribe/out.

10 Foster S. (2017). 'The benefits of values-based recruitment'. *British Journal of Nursing*, 26(10), p. 579. https://doi.org/10.12968/bjon.2017.26.10.579.

11 Miller, S.L. (2015). 'Values-based recruitment in health care'. *Nursing Standard*, 29(21), pp. 37–41.

12 Newman, A., Donohue, R., & Eva, N. (2017). 'Psychological safety: A systematic review of the literature'. *Human Resource Management Review*, 27(3), pp. 521–535. https://doi.org/10.1016/j.hrmr.2017.001.001.

13 Newdick, C., & Danbury, C. (2015). 'Culture, compassion and clinical neglect: probity in the NHS after Mid Staffordshire'. *Journal of Medical Ethics*, 41(12), pp. 956–962. https://doi.org/10.1136/medethics-2012-101048.

15   The Culture Club

1   Kegan, R., Lahey, L., Miller, M.L., Fleming, A. & Helsing, D. (2016). *An everyone culture: Becoming a deliberately developmental organization.* Harvard Business Review Press.

2   Zenger, J. & Folkman, J. (2013, March 15). 'The ideal praise-to-criticism ratio'. *Harvard Business Review.* https://hbr.org/2013/03/the-ideal-praise-to-criticism.

16   Telling our stories

1   Bhugra, D., & Jones, P. (2001). 'Migration and mental illness'. *Advances in Psychiatric Treatment*, 7(3), pp. 216–222. doi:10.1192/apt.7.3.216.

2   McKellar, D., Renner, D., Gower, A., O'Brien, S., Stevens, A., DiNiro, A. (2020). 'Everyone matters; everyone contributes; everyone grows: a pilot project cultivating psychological safety to promote growth-oriented service culture after the Oakden Report'. *Australian Health Review* 44, pp. 867–872. https://doi.org/10.1071/AH20156.

17 Trauma and transformation

1   Cooney, A., & O'Shea, E. (2019). 'The impact of life story work on person-centred care for people with dementia living in long-stay care settings in Ireland'. *Dementia, 18*(7–8), 2731–2746. https://doi.org/10.1177/1471301218756123. Accessed 25 September 2021.

2   Clinical Excellence Commission. (2014). *TOP 5: Improving the care of patients with dementia 2012–2013.* Clinical Excellence Commission. https://www.cec.health.nsw.gov.au/__data/assets/pdf_file/0006/268215/TOP5-Final-Report.pdf. Accessed 25 September 2021.

3   Van der Kolk, B. (2014). *The body keeps the score. Mind, brain and body in the transformation of trauma.* Penguin Books.

4   Lloyd, P. (Director). (2008). *Mamma Mia!* [Film]. Littlestar Productions & Playtone.

18 It all comes together

1   Key, K.H. (2018). *Foundations of Trauma-Informed Care: An Introductory Primer.* LeadingAge. https://www.leadingage.org/sites/default/files/RFA%20Primer%20_%20RGB.pdf.

2   Felitti, V.J., Anda, R.F., Nordenberg, D., Williamson, D.F., Spitz, A.M., Edwards, V., Koss, M.P., & Marks, J.S. (1998). 'Relationship of childhood abuse and household dysfunction to many of the leading causes of death in adults. The Adverse Childhood Experiences (ACE) Study'. *American Journal of Preventive Medicine, 14*(4), pp. 245–258. https://doi.org/10.1016/s0749-3797(98)00017-8.

3   Substance Abuse and Mental Health Services Administration. (2014). *SAMHSA's Concept of Trauma and Guidance for a Trauma-Informed Approach.* HHS Publication No. (SMA) 14-4884. Substance Abuse and Mental Health Services Administration. https://ncsacw.samhsa.gov/userfiles/files/SAMHSA_Trauma.pdf.

4   Key, K.H. (2018). *Foundations of Trauma-Informed Care: An Introductory Primer.* LeadingAge. https://www.leadingage.org/sites/default/files/RFA%20Primer%20_%20RGB.pdf.

5   Moreno-Morales, C., Calero, R., Moreno-Morales, P., & Pintado, C. (2020). 'Music therapy in the treatment of dementia: a systematic review and meta-analysis'. *Frontiers in medicine, 7,* p. 160. https://www.frontiersin.org/articles/10.3389/fmed.2020.00160/full?report=reader.

6   Garrido, S., Dunne, L., Chang, E., Perz, J., Stevens, C.J., & Haertsch, M. (2017). 'The Use of Music Playlists for People with Dementia: A Critical Synthesis'. *Journal of Alzheimer's Disease, 60*(3), pp. 1129–1142. https://doi.org/10.3233/JAD-170612.

7   Gaviola, M.A., Inder, K.J., Dilworth, S., Holliday, E.G., & Higgins, I. (2020). 'Impact of individualised music listening intervention on persons with dementia: A systematic review of randomised controlled trials'. *Australasian Journal on Ageing, 39*(1), pp. 10–20. https://doi.org/10.1111/ajag.12642.

19 Burning down and burning out

1   Heinemann, L.V., & Heinemann, T. (2017). 'Burnout research: Emergence and scientific investigation of a contested diagnosis.' *Sage Open, 7*(1). https://doi.org/10.1177%2F2158244017697154.

2   Giorgi, G., Arcangeli, G., Perminiene, M., Lorini, C., Ariza-Montes, A., Fiz-Perez, J., Di Fabio, A., & Mucci, N. (2017). 'Work-Related Stress in the Banking Sector: A Review of Incidence, Correlated Factors, and Major Consequences'. *Frontiers in Psychology, 8,* p. 2166. https://doi.org/10.3389/fpsyg.2017.02166.

3   Blanding, M. (2015, January 15). 'National Health Costs Could Decrease if Managers Reduce Work Stress, Harvard Business School.' *Working Knowledge.* https://hbswk.hbs.edu/item/national-health-costs-could-decrease-if-managers-reduce-work-stress.

Notes

4   Medibank Private. (2008). 'The Cost of Workplace Stress in Australia'. https://www.
     medibank.com.au/client/documents/pdfs/the-cost-of-workplace-stress.pdf.

5   Toppinen-Tanner, S., Ahola, K., Koskinen, A., & Väänänen, A. (2009). 'Burnout
     predicts hospitalization for mental and cardiovascular disorders: 10-year
     prospective results from industrial sector'. *Stress and Health: Journal of the
     International Society for the Investigation of Stress*, 25(4), pp. 287–296. https://doi.
     org/10.1002/smi.1282.

6   Ahola, K. (2007). *Occupational burnout and health (People and work research reports,
     81)*. Helsinki: Finnish Institute of Occupational Health.

7   Bakker, A.B., Le Blanc, P.M., & Schaufeli, W.B. (2005). 'Burnout contagion among
     intensive care nurses'. *Journal of Advanced Nursing*, 51(3), 276–287. https://doi.
     org/10.1111/j.1365-2648.2005.03494.x.

8   González-Morales, M.G., Peiró, J.M., Rodríguez, I., & Bliese, P.D. (2012). 'Perceived
     collective burnout: a multilevel explanation of burnout'. *Anxiety, Stress, and Coping*,
     25(1), pp. 43–61. https://doi.org/10.1080/10615806.2010.542808.

9   Maslach, C., & Leiter, M.P. (2016). 'Understanding the burnout experience: recent
     research and its implications for psychiatry'. *World psychiatry: Official Journal of
     the World Psychiatric Association (WPA)*, 15(2), pp. 103–111. https://doi.org/10.1002/
     wps.20311.

10   Maslach, C., & Leiter, M.P. (2016). 'Understanding the burnout experience: recent
     research and its implications for psychiatry'. *World Psychiatry: Official Journal of
     the World Psychiatric Association (WPA)*, 15(2), pp. 103–111. https://doi.org/10.1002/
     wps.20311.

11   Leiter, M.P., Laschinger, H., Day, A., & Oore, D.G. (2011). 'The impact of civility
     interventions on employee social behavior, distress, and attitudes'. *Journal of Applied
     Psychology*, 96(6), pp. 1258–1274. https://doi.org/10.1037/a0024442.

12   Palmer, P.J. (2000). *Let your life speak: Listening for the voice of vocation*. Jossey-Bass.

13   *ibid.*

20 On being story-informed

1   Kegan, R., Lahey, L., Miller, M.L., Fleming, A. & Helsing, D. (2016). *An everyone
     culture: Becoming a deliberately developmental organization*. Harvard Business Review
     Press.

2   Gawande, A. (2014). *Being mortal: Medicine and what matters in the end*. Metropolitan
     Books/Henry Holt and Company.

3   Charon, R. (2006). *Narrative Medicine: Honoring the stories of illness*. Oxford
     University Press.

4   Ensign J. (2014, July 16). 'The problem(s) with narrative medicine'. *Josphine
     Ensign Medical Margins: On Humanizing Health Care*. https://josephineensign.
     com/2014/07/16/the-problems-with-narrative-medicine/

5   Riess, H. (2018). *The empathy effect: Seven neuroscience-based key for transforming the
     way we live, love, work, and connect across differences*. Sounds True.

6   Merriam-Webster. *Equality*. https://www.merriam-webster.com/dictionary/equality.
     Accessed 25 September 2021.

7   Equality and Human Rights Commission. (2018). 'Understanding equality.'
     https://www.equalityhumanrights.com/en/secondary-education-resources/
     useful-information/understanding-equality.

8   D'Souza, S. & Renner, D. (2014). *Not knowing: The art of turning uncertainty into
     opportunity*. LID Publishing.

9   Romans 12:3. *Holy Bible: New Living Translation*. (2004). Tyndale House Publishers.

10   Philippians 2:3-4. *Holy Bible: New Living Translation*. (2004). Tyndale House
     Publishers.

11   Foster, N. (Host). (December 15, 2020). Lacy Borgo – Holding centre. *Renovaré Podcast* Episode 198. [Audio podcast]. ttps://renovare.org/podcast/lacy-borgo-holding-center.

12   Novy, C. (2018). 'Life stories and their performance in dementia care'. *The Arts in Psychotherapy.* 57: 95–101. https://doi.org/10.1016/j.aip.2017.12.003.

13   Qadar, S. (Presenter/Host). (2007). 'Deep listening: Working with Indigenous mental distress'. *All in the mind* [Radio program]. Guest speakers D. McDermott, C. Byrne, R. Lowe, W. Nolan, D. Parkinson, J. Punch. ABC Radio National.

14   Gawande, A. (2014). *Being mortal: Medicine and what matters in the end.* Metropolitan Books/Henry Holt and Company.

15   Covey, S.R. (1989). *The seven habits of highly effective people: Restoring the character ethic.* Simon and Schuster.

16   Coles, R. (1989). *The call of stories: Teaching and the moral imagination.* Houghton, Mifflin and Company.

17   Saturday Night Live. (2013, September 21). Today show: Everyone has a story – Saturday Night Live. https://www.youtube.com/watch?v=-k-BZKQpCRk.

18   Kusmaul, N. & Anderson, K. (2018). 'Applying a trauma-informed perspective to loss and change in the lives of older adults'. *Social Work in Health Care*, 57(5), pp. 355–375. doi: 10.1080/00981389.2018.1447531.

19   Bardsley, A. & Morgan, S. (2021). 'Final picture of couple married for 70 years who died days apart with Covid.' *Wales Online.* https://www.walesonline.co.uk/news/uk-news/final-picture-couple-married-70-19800234.

Gratitude

Sincere thanks to Julia Beaven and Michael Bollen from Wakefield Press for recognising that *An Everyone Story* has something to add to the world. Julia, your encouragement and editorial support has been tremendously meaningful to me. Special thanks also to my good friend Vicki Jacobs – who needs a literary agent with you around?

Writing a coherent manuscript in crevices wedged between the demands of life and work is a long haul. I couldn't have done it without the editorial support of Georgia Laval and Kit Carstairs (from The Manuscript Appraisal Agency) or my beta readers – especially Christine Beal, Stephen Judd, and Deej Eszenyi – your candour made all the difference. Thank you also to John Swinton, Sue Kurrle, Kim Manley, Colm Cunningham and Jason van Genderen for your generous endorsement of this work.

Thank you, Leon Pericles, for sharing your remarkable work, *Islands of Lost Memories*, as the companion image for this book. You demonstrate the power of art to succinctly capture something that has taken me thousands of words to say.

Barb Spriggs, thank you for sharing your story, for becoming my ally in bringing this book to fruition and for your wonderful warm smiles.

Thank you, Aaron Groves: when you asked me to join your team, I did not anticipate that the experience would change me and how I see the world, but it did. Thank you also to my colleagues from the

Oakden Review panel, Del Thomson and Nicholas Procter. It was a privilege to work alongside you.

Thank you, Sujeeve Sanmuganatham, for asking me to help in the mayhem after the report's publication. Thank you, Jackie Hanson and Scott McMullen, for giving me space to lead and for going on the journey of transformation together. Thank you, Tom Stubbs, for your outstanding leadership of the Oakden Oversight Committee, I learnt a lot from watching you at work.

Thank you also to the team of very special people who came together in those early, challenging days after the Oakden Report, and to the remarkable team at Northgate House. I've told many of your stories across the pages of this book – thank you for believing that we could find a better way to come to work. For an interim service, Northgate House has punched above its weight. It was never intended to continue indefinitely in its temporary digs. Whatever the future holds, the stories from residents, families and staff are precious and offer lessons worthy of attention.

Thank you, Andrew Stevens and Uncharted Leadership – serendipity, indeed! I value every conversation with you. Our mutual learning and growth have been gifts. Thank you to Heidi Silverston and Amelia Gower from the South Australian Department of Health and Wellbeing for your faithful support of the growth culture project. Thank you also to Penny Joyes in the Office of the Chief Psychiatrist for valiantly advocating for the mental health and wellbeing of older people. Thank you, John Brayley, Chief Psychiatrist, for your support and for putting the person before the system.

As 2021 drew to a close, I sensed another vocational stirring. I took the heart-wrenching step of moving on from my work in the South Australian Department of Health and Wellbeing, precipitated by an exciting opportunity for my wife Lois to take a new job in Scotland – the land of my ancestors. Concurrently, the opportunity arose for me to join the wonderful team at The Dementia Centre, HammondCare, working with the Australian and international teams. Thank you to the team at HammondCare – Mike Baird, Angela Raguz, Colm

Cunningham, Marie Alford and the amazing, values-driven team across all corners of the organisation – for welcoming me. *An Everyone Story* aligns exactly with our mission in action.

Lastly, thank you to my family. To my father, I am grateful for the years we have had to grow together. Your life leaves a legacy. To my three talented and beautiful girls, Elspeth, Erin and Edie: I'm proud of you as three strong women taking the next generational journey for our family. She hardly had time to know you, but your grandmother, Lizzy, loved you deeply. Thank you, Lois. You are the best person I know. Your love and acceptance have been the most potent source of strength for me for many years. I love you.

www.ingramcontent.com/pod-product-compliance
Lightning Source LLC
Chambersburg PA
CBHW040147270326
41929CB00025B/3409